Learning Strategies:
Your Guide to Classroom and Test-Taking Success
First Edition

Editor

Amanda Wolkowitz, PhD
Psychometrician
Assessment Technologies Institute®, LLC

Associate Editors

Tony Juve, PhD
Psychometrician

Matthew Scaruto, MA
Research Associate

Johanna Barnes, BA Journalism
Product Developer

Preface

Learning Strategies: Your Guide to Classroom and Test-Taking Success is a research-based book designed to help you prepare for the college classroom and improve your academic performance.

The book begins with self-assessment inventories that will help you quickly determine your strengths and weaknesses inside and outside the classroom. They will also provide a general assessment of your test-taking skills. The remainder of the book provides strategies for absorbing more information during lectures, creating and maintaining productive study environments, and succeeding on classroom and standardized tests.

After the inventories in Chapter 1, Chapters 2 to 7 of this book are structured similarly. Each chapter is divided into sections. At the beginning of each section, research is presented about a learning or test-taking strategy. This is followed by a list of hands-on strategies. At the end of each section are application exercises of the strategies as well as a summary and a set of review problems. The solutions to the review problems are at the end of the book.

table of contents

This chapter contains six self-assessment inventories. Complete each of these inventories to determine which chapters in this book will benefit you most. These inventories are meant as a guide. Even if you do well, you may still benefit from some of the strategies presented in each chapter.

Inventory 1: Getting the Most from Lectures

Read the following statements. Mark the statements with which you agree.

- ☐ I often refer to the class objectives on the syllabus.
- ☐ I usually have my reading assignments completed before lecture.
- ☐ I only miss one or two classes, if any, per semester.
- ☐ Most of my learning occurs outside of lecture.
- ☐ I come to class with questions about the material.
- ☐ I usually write down information from the text as I read.
- ☐ I am comfortable with my note-taking strategies.
- ☐ I use a template for taking notes.
- ☐ I do not write down everything the instructor writes or displays.
- ☐ I am able to stay focused during the entire lecture.
- ☐ I do not outline my notes as I take them in class.
- ☐ I am not concerned about spelling or grammar mistakes in my notes.
- ☐ I write down information that the instructor says, but does not write or display.
- ☐ I find it useful to write examples in my notes.
- ☐ I keep my notes organized.

Count the number of check marks and use the following rubric as a guide to assess your ability to get the most from lectures.

NUMBER OF CHECK MARKS	RESULT
15	You are getting the most from lectures.
13 – 14	You are learning quite a bit from lecture, but you may benefit from a few strategies in Chapter 2.
9 – 12	While you are following some strategies for getting the most out of lecture, there are several strategies that could help you get even more out of class. Refer to Chapter 2.
0 – 8	You are not getting the most out of lecture. Refer to Chapter 2 for ways to benefit more from lecture.

Inventory 2: Everyday Learning

Read the following statements. Mark the statements with which you agree.

- ☐ I study in settings similar to those in which I first learned the information.
- ☐ My study environment has few distractions.
- ☐ I know at what point during the day my alertness and energy levels are at their highest.
- ☐ I am able to complete all of my reading assignments on time.
- ☐ I skim each reading assignment to get the main idea before reading the assignment in detail.
- ☐ I have techniques for comprehending and remembering what I have read.
- ☐ I know the difference between visual, tactile, and auditory learners.
- ☐ I know my preferred learning styles.
- ☐ I use several learning strategies that complement my learning style.
- ☐ I know whether I am a reflective learner or an active learner.
- ☐ I know whether I am a concrete or abstract thinker.
- ☐ I know there are different types of intelligences.
- ☐ I know my multiple intelligences.
- ☐ I have strategies that complement my multiple intelligences.
- ☐ I use mnemonic devices to help me remember definitions and formulas.
- ☐ It is easy for me to memorize facts.
- ☐ I am good at remembering the spelling and definition of words.

Count the number of check marks and use the following rubric as a guide to assess your everyday learning strategies.

NUMBER OF CHECK MARKS	RESULT
16 – 17	You know your learning style and complementary learning strategies.
13 – 15	You are familiar with learning styles and strategies, but you may benefit from the information provided in Chapter 3.
9 – 12	You have some knowledge about learning styles and strategies; however, there is more you could learn that could help you in class. Refer to Chapter 3.
0 – 8	You do not know your learning style. Refer to Chapter 3 for ways to identify your learning styles and for strategies to complement your style.

Inventory 3: Purpose of Assessments

Read the following statements. Mark the statements with which you agree.

☐ Tests can be subclassified as classroom or standardized.

☐ Classroom tests typically use a greater variety of item types (e.g., true/false, short answer, performance tasks, and multiple-choice) than do standardized tests.

☐ Classroom tests are well-suited for measuring student progress on specific course outcomes.

☐ Classroom tests help teachers make teaching decisions.

☐ Standardized tests are well-suited for making comparisons across large groups of people.

☐ I may be able to obtain a list of objectives for a standardized test.

☐ There are different ways that multiple-choice questions can be scored.

☐ It is important to know the format of a test ahead of time.

☐ Standardized and classroom assessments differ in the way they are developed.

Count the number of check marks and use the following rubric as a guide to assess your level of understanding of classroom and standardized tests.

NUMBER OF CHECK MARKS	RESULT
8 – 9	You have a good understanding of classroom and standardized tests.
6 – 7	You have a fair understanding of classroom and standardized tests. You may benefit from the information provided in Chapter 4.
0 – 5	You have a lot to learn about classroom and standardized tests. Review Chapter 4.

Inventory 4: Before the Test

Read the following statements. Mark the statements with which you agree.

☐ I understand the difference between a recall and recognition test.

☐ I know the format of the test before taking it.

☐ I know the purpose of the test before taking it.

☐ I usually start studying at least two weeks before a test.

☐ I rarely stay up late the night before a test.

☐ I study alone and with peers.

☐ I set aside time for studying and stick to that schedule.

☐ I set goals for my studying.

☐ I answer practice questions during my study sessions.

☐ I always eat a good breakfast the morning of an exam.

☐ I dress in layers or bring extra clothes to a test.

☐ I know what type of snacks will give my body and brain enough energy to take a test.

☐ I do not review test material with peers immediately before taking a test.

Count the number of check marks and use the following rubric as a guide to assess your ability to prepare for a test.

NUMBER OF CHECK MARKS	RESULT
13	You are preparing well for the test.
11 – 12	You have some good strategies for studying for a test, but you may benefit from a few strategies Chapter 5 has to offer.
8 – 10	While you are following some test preparation strategies, there are several study strategies that could help you prepare even better. Refer to Chapter 5.
0 – 7	You are not preparing for a test in the best way. Refer to Chapter 5 for study strategies.

Inventory 5: During the Test

Read the following statements. Mark the statements with which you agree.

- ☐ I usually take time to relax before and during an exam.
- ☐ I use a watch to pace myself during exams.
- ☐ I quickly review tests before budgeting my testing time.
- ☐ I usually read the directions before starting a test.
- ☐ I have experience taking multiple-choice tests.
- ☐ I ask the instructor if I'm unclear about a question or the directions on a test.
- ☐ If I don't know an answer to a test question, I make an educated guess.
- ☐ I rule out implausible distractors when selecting a correct answer.
- ☐ I look for relationships in the item stem and response choices when selecting answers.
- ☐ I have experience taking essay tests.
- ☐ I use brief outlines during an essay test to organize and clarify my thoughts.
- ☐ I keep my essay responses brief, but explain statements and support ideas with facts.
- ☐ I typically use short, simple sentences to make arguments in essay tests.
- ☐ I am familiar with common verbs used in essay questions.
- ☐ I am concerned about my handwriting, spelling, and grammar during essay exams.
- ☐ I include introductions or thesis statements in my essays.
- ☐ I use summaries and conclusions in my essays.
- ☐ I use transitional words when composing essays to improve the clarity of my writing.
- ☐ I use headings, numbering, or spacing to clearly communicate when composing essays.
- ☐ I proofread my essay exams before submitting them to the instructor.

Count the number of check marks and use the following rubric as a guide to assess your test-taking strategies.

NUMBER OF CHECK MARKS	RESULT
18 – 20	You're using most of the recommended test-taking strategies.
12 – 17	You're using some good test-taking strategies, but you may benefit from a few more strategies discussed in Chapter 6.
6 – 11	You're following some important test-taking strategies, but you could improve more by reviewing Chapter 6.
0 – 5	You're not really using recommended test-taking strategies. Take some time to review the strategies in Chapter 6.

Inventory 6: After the Test

Read the following statements. Mark the statements with which you agree.

☐ My test grades reflect what I know.

☐ I know which study strategies work for me and which do not.

☐ I have found a way to balance my work schedule and my studying.

☐ My test anxiety does not affect my test performance.

☐ I take a break immediately after taking a test.

☐ I review information that was on the test periodically throughout the rest of the semester.

☐ I read any feedback my instructor writes on my test.

☐ I always look at the mistakes I made on my test and figure out the correct answer.

Count the number of check marks and use the following rubric as a guide to assess your ability to retain information learned from a test.

NUMBER OF CHECK MARKS	RESULT
8	You know how to study and retain the information learned from a test.
6 – 7	You have some good strategies to implement after taking a test, but you may benefit from a few strategies Chapter 7 has to offer.
5	While you have some good ideas of ways to learn from and retain information after taking a test, there are several additional strategies that you may want to consider. Refer to Chapter 7.
0 – 4	There are strategies for retaining and learning from your test. You are not benefiting from these strategies. Refer to Chapter 7 for some helpful tips.

Listening to instructors lecture is part of the learning experience. Lectures can be given in a traditional classroom or online. Regardless of the mode of presentation, being a successful student involves getting the most from these lectures. This chapter will discuss ways to prepare for class and strategies for getting the most from lectures, including note-taking strategies.

2.1 Preparing for class

How do you prepare for class? Do you read assignments before class? Do you complete your written homework? Do you show up to lecture on time and ready to learn? If you want to get the most out of any lecture, you should understand that preparing for class is more than just completing written assignments. Preparing for class means reading the assigned text, studying on a regular basis, and coming to class ready to learn. Research has shown that most of the learning during a semester does not come from listening to an instructor talk during lecture, but from preparing for class (Jacobs & Hyman, 2006). During a lecture, the instructor's role is to explain concepts, highlight important topics, and answer questions. Your role is to come to class prepared so that you can get the most out of the explained concepts, fill in the details of important topics, and get questions answered. The information in this section can help you get the most out of lectures by providing tips on ways to prepare for class. This section will offer strategies for preparing for class by providing you with information related to the following questions:

- How do I prepare for a lecture?

- How do I get the most out of class during a lecture?

How do I prepare for a lecture?

Preparing for class not only means that you attend class and stay alert during the lecture, but it also means that you are coming to class with assignments completed and prepared to take notes. It may be tempting to only complete assignments that you have to hand in for a grade, but it is just as important to complete reading assignments. Research has shown that most students do not read the assigned material before class (Burchfield & Sapington, 2000; Clump, Bauer, & Bradley, 2004). Research has also shown that students who take the time to read and then answer a set of questions related to the readings or write summaries of the readings will be more involved in lectures than those students who fail to complete the assigned material (Carney, Fry, Gabriele, & Ballard, 2008).

 Hands-on strategies

The following list of strategies offers some tips for preparing for a lecture.

- **Read the class outline and objectives.** The objectives identify the major topics that will be presented in class.

- **Compare assigned text to class objectives.** The text most closely aligned with the class objectives indicates key areas to study.

- **Preview the chapter.** Look at the chapter and read the section headings to identify the content being covered.

- **Read the required reading before class.** Make brief notes in your own words. Your goal is to get a general understanding of the material. Don't get bogged down in difficult sections. After all, you haven't heard the lecture yet.

- **Write down questions to ask in class.** As you read through the readings, write down any questions or concepts that are unclear. Make sure you get your questions answered during lecture.

- **Review the chapter quickly before class.** A quick review of the chapter or your notes will help you focus on the material and help jog your memory of the concepts and any questions that arose as you prepared for lecture.

How do I get the most out of class during a lecture?

Being prepared for lecture means not only completing assignments, but also being prepared to take notes during lecture. Before class, make sure you know the mode of presentation your instructor prefers. Many instructors choose to use some form of electronic notes, such as PowerPoint presentations. Teachers choose these modes of presentation to cover more material and reduce the amount of information that must be written on a chalkboard or whiteboard (Pardini, Domizi, Forbes, & Pettis, 2005). If your instructor uses electronic notes, find out if you can print these notes before lecture and use them as a starting point for your in-class notes. If your instructor uses more traditional modes of presentation, be prepared with a pen or pencil, paper, and perhaps a template for note-taking. As explained in the next section (2.2 Taking notes), students who are prepared and take good notes during lecture tend to perform better in class than students ill-prepared for note-taking (Peverly et al, 2007; Terry, 2006; Titsworth & Kiewra, 2004; Williams & Eggert, 2005).

Hands-on strategies

The following list of strategies offers some tips for getting the most out of class during a lecture.

- **Attend class.** If you don't attend class, you will not get anything out of the lecture. If you must miss class, let the instructor know and be sure to get notes from someone in class who you know takes good notes.

- **Sit near the front of the class.** Imagine the instructor is speaking just to you.

- **Change seats every now and then, and avoid sitting near friends.** You are less likely to become distracted and miss important information if you don't have a friend next to you.

- **Focus on the content, not the instructor's characteristics or mannerisms.** You are less likely to miss some important part of the lecture if you are properly focused.

- **Be alert for repetition of concepts.** Important concepts may be repeated using various methods. Be alert for words or phrases such as "remember," "the most important," and "as stated before," and note when an instructor emphasizes a concept by providing an example of how it is applied.

- **Take good notes.** Taking good notes requires practice. See the next section in this chapter for good note-taking strategies.

 Applications

1. Review the excerpt from a chemistry syllabus below. What are the major topics you could expect during lectures on this chapter? Are there any sections from the textbook that the instructor is not going to cover? What are the reading and homework assignments? When are they due? Do the assignments coincide with the lecture topics?

CHAPTER 3: PERIODIC TABLE LECTURE TOPICS	DATE	ASSIGNMENT	COMMENTS
3.1 Introduction and History of the Periodic Table	March 1	Read 3.1 to 3.2	
3.2 Nuclear Charge of Atoms	March 2-5	3.2 #5-12; Read 3.3	
3.3 Molar Mass of Atoms	March 8	3.3 #1-10; Read 3.4	Quiz over 3.1, 3.2
3.4 Ions	March 9	3.4 #2, 6, 9-15; Read 3.5	
3.5 Ionization Energy	March 10	3.5 #1, 3, 5-10; Read 3.7	
3.7 Electron Affinity	March 11-12	Write 5 review questions	
Review	March 15		
Test	March 16		Test over Chapter 3 Chapter 3 homework due

Possible response: If you were taking this chemistry class, you would expect to learn about the history of the periodic table during the first lecture. You would realize that your instructor will spend two weeks on the chapter, but plans to skip section 3.6. This syllabus also clearly indicates the assignments related to the lecture topics and shows that you will have a quiz on March 8, a test on March 16, and your homework will be due the day of the test.

2. Preview Chapter 3 of this book. Based on the headings and subheadings, what do you expect to learn in this chapter? Write down your expectations and then read Chapter 3. Were your expectations met? Was it helpful?

3. When reading text to prepare for class, it may be helpful to highlight, outline or diagram key points. Also, use the margins to write down questions. Try highlighting, outlining, or diagramming the paragraph below. Write down any questions. Do you find one method better than another? Examples of each of these techniques are shown below; however, if you prefer a different method of outlining or diagramming, then you should use that method.

> Avogadro's number
>
> In chemistry, a unit called a **mole** is often used to discuss the quantity of a substance. A mole is 6.02×10^{23} representative particles of a substance (that is, atoms, molecules or other units). This particular number was found experimentally by Amedeo Avogadro di Quaregna and is called Avogadro's number in his honor. The mass in grams of a substance is the **molar mass** of substance. Calculations in terms of moles are often done in chemistry.

Example:

Highlight/Underline:

> Avogadro's number
>
> In chemistry, a unit called a **mole** is often used to discuss the quantity of a substance. <u>A mole is 6.02×10^{23} representative particles of a substance</u> (that is, atoms, molecules or other units). This particular number was found experimentally by Amedeo Avogadro di Quaregna and is called <u>Avogadro's number</u> in his honor. The mass in grams of a substance is the **molar mass** of substance. Calculations in terms of moles are often done in chemistry.

Outline:

A. Avogadro's number
  1. 1 mole = 6.02×10^{23} particles
  2. used to calculate molar mass of a substance

Questions:

What is an example calculation?

Do I need to memorize this value?

How was this number determined?

Diagram:

Avogadro's number

1 mole

6.02×10^{23} particles

used to calculate molar mass of a substance

4. A friend of yours is struggling in a science class. You know that she attends class regularly and tends to sit in the back of the room by the door. She also writes down everything the teacher says in her notes. What strategies might you offer to her so that she could improve her performance in the class?

Possible response: It's great that she attends the class, but perhaps she should try sitting in different areas of the classroom, including the front of the room. By sitting near the front of the room, she may be able to focus more on the content being presented and be more alert for concepts that the teacher repeats. By being more focused during class, her notes may also become a better source for review.

Summary

Succeeding in a course involves preparing for lectures and capitalizing on your time in lecture. Preparing for lecture means completing all assignments, including assigned readings. Although you may not read chapters in great detail before a lecture, you should be familiar with the material that your instructor presents. The more prepared you are for lecture, the more you will learn. If you have done all the appropriate preparatory work, don't forget the other practical strategies for getting the most out of lecture, such as changing seats occasionally and focusing on the content.

Review

Select the best response for questions 1 and 2. Provide a response for question 3. Answers are provided at the end of this book.

1. Most of the learning during a lecture takes place while doing which of the following tasks?

    A. Completing assigned material before lecture

    B. Reviewing assigned readings immediately before lecture

    C. Listening during lecture

    D. Asking questions during lecture

2. True   False   Most students complete the assigned reading before lecture.

3. List three strategies that may help enhance your learning during a lecture.

    1. _____

    2. _____

    3. _____

2.2 Taking notes

Do you ever wonder what to write down during lecture? Should you write down everything the instructor says or writes? If the instructor lectures directly from the text, is it necessary to rewrite that information in your notes? Taking notes during lecture may seem trivial to some; however, research has shown that students who are able to take high-quality notes tend to perform better on assessments related to lecture material than those who are poor note-takers (Peverly et al., 2007; Terry, 2006; Titsworth & Kiewra, 2004; Williams & Eggert, 2005). This chapter will offer note-taking strategies that may help your performance in class by answering the following questions:

- What information should I write down?

- How do I organize my notes during lecture?

What information should I write down?

Do you write down everything the instructor writes down during lecture? Do you ever write down more than what the instructor writes down? Do you ever write down less? You may be surprised to find out that you don't need to write down everything the instructor writes. Keep in mind that your instructor will probably explain information discussed in your textbook or other assigned text. Your instructor may also present the same idea in several ways or in several examples. You do not need to write down all of these explanations, but you do need to be able to distinguish key concepts that the instructor is trying to help you understand. (Williams & Eggert, 2005; Titsworth & Kiewra, 2004).

For example, how many times have you been in class when a question was posed to the instructor about information coming directly from the text? Similarly, how many times have you been in class when a question was posed to the instructor about information that didn't exist in the textbook, but was related to the topic? In the first situation, if the answer is clearly written in the assigned reading, it is not necessary to repeat the information in your lecture notes. In the second situation, however, it is important to write down the answer provided by the instructor because it may help clarify difficult concepts and it is not available in your assigned readings. If you fail to write down the question and answer from these types of scenarios, as many students do (Baker & Lombardi, 1985; Kiewra, DuBois, Christian & McShane, 1988; O'Donnell & Dansereau, 1993), then you are not getting the most out of lecture.

 Hands-on Strategies

The following list of suggestions may help you develop strategies toward becoming a better note-taker.

- **Be a good listener.** By being an active listener in lecture, you will likely write more meaningful notes and get more out of lecture.

- **Capture unfamiliar information.** It is not important to write down everything the instructor says, but be alert for new information.

- **Be as brief as possible.** Your lecture notes are not the place to write long prose. Keep them brief so that you can capture more.

- **It is not necessary to write down information that is directly taken from your textbook, such as definitions.** You may want to have your textbook open to the section being covered in lecture so you know what presented information is directly from the book.

- **Write down examples that help explain or reinforce a concept.** If you don't write it down, you may not remember it when you need it.

- **Don't try to outline your notes during lecture.** This is not a good use of your lecture time. You can outline later if you wish.

- **Don't worry about spelling or grammar — unless the lesson is on one of these topics.** Your notes are for you. They do not need to follow spelling and grammar rules.

- **If you had questions related to the material before lecture, be sure to ask them and write down the answers.** Lecture is usually a good time to ask your instructor questions related to the material.

How do I organize my notes during lecture?

Do you have a method for taking notes in class? Do you find your notes unorganized when you review them? Do you use different techniques for note-taking depending on how your instructor lectures? Your instructor may present a lecture in a variety of ways. He or she may use a chalk or dry-erase board, PowerPoint, or may simply lecture without visual aids. Regardless of the instructional method, being a good note-taker means that you can adapt your note-taking strategies to fit the method used by your instructor. Since most of a student's time in class is spent listening to the instructor lecture (as opposed to spending class time to take a test or do group work) and most collegiate faculty use the lecture format as their preferred instructional method (Armbruster, 2009; Wirt et al., 2001), it is important to know how to set up and organize your notes for a variety of lecture formats. In addition, having organized notes will help you review the lecture information at a later time (Terry, 2006).

 Hands-on Strategies

The following strategies may help you organize your notes for any type of lecture format.

- **Use a template for note-taking.**

- **Use a separate folder or notebook for each subject.**

- **Be prepared to take notes for the lecture format used by your instructor** (e.g., traditional lecture or guided web notes).

- **Start with enough clean paper, pen/pencil, or other materials you may need to get you through class.** You shouldn't bother other students during lecture by ruffling through your bag to get supplies or asking someone next to you for extra paper. It's a distraction for you, too.

- **Date and title your notes.** Use section and subsection headings.

- **Write legibly or use a computer.** If you use shorthand, make sure you remember the meaning of the symbols and abbreviations in your shorthand.

- **Leave wide margins, extra lines at the end of each section, or double space your notes**. This will allow you to fill in missing or pertinent information at a later time.

- **Consider writing on one side of the paper only.** It is easier to read notes when writing does not show through the paper.

 Applications

1. One of your friends is having trouble keeping up with the pace of a biology lecture. He complains that the instructor goes through the PowerPoint slides too quickly for students to write down the information. He also complains that the instructor just reiterates the information provided in the textbook (sometimes verbatim) and that he never has time to ask a question because he's writing so furiously. What suggestions could you offer to him?

Possible response: First, see if you can print the PowerPoint slides ahead of time. If not, make sure you read the material before lecture and only write down the information not provided in the text. You can go back and take notes from the text outside of lecture time. By not taking unnecessary notes, you will have more time to ask questions and write down the answers.

2. Note-taking templates can be a good way to organize your notes during a lecture. An example of a note-taking template is shown below. In addition, two blank templates are also displayed. During the next lecture, try using one of these templates or make one up for yourself. You may be surprised at how much it helps you stay focused and organized during lecture. When using one of these templates, be sure to keep the notes for a certain class all together in one binder, write legibly (or type), and consider using only one side of the paper.

Example

Science	(Date)	Page 1
Insects		
I. Body Parts	Insects have 3 body parts: head, body, thorax	
	Head: one pair of antennae and 3 pairs of mouth parts	
	Thorax includes 3 pairs of legs (and wings)	
	Abdomen can have 11 segments – reproductive parts usually on segments 8, 9, 10	
II. Mouth Parts	Mouth is adaptable to different types of food – some are chewing, piercing, sucking	
III. Legs and Wings	Wings and legs also adapted for swift locomotion	
	Some are aquatic, burrowing, running, flying	
	Some have lost their legs from lack of movement	

Subject	Date	Page

Concept		Key Points

Summary

Lectures are one of the most common ways instructors provide information to you and you will spend a great deal of time taking notes. Because research has demonstrated that student lecture notes are often incomplete or inaccurate, this chapter has provided you with suggestions on how to get the most out of lecture and take better notes. Chapter 3 will focus on how to use these notes and other everyday learning strategies to be successful in class.

Review

Determine whether the statements are true or false. Select the correct response. Answers are provided at the end of this book.

1. True   False   Research indicates that academic performance is positively correlated with the quality of notes a student takes in class.

2. True   False   It is important to try to record all of the information an instructor presents during a lecture.

3. True   False   Studies have shown that less than half of university professors use lecture format as their primary instructional method.

4. True   False   The note-taking process should begin before arriving at class.

5. True   False   Outlining notes during lecture will help students better retain information.

6. True   False   Students should only take notes on material they understand; taking notes on material they do not understand could cause the notes to be confusing.

References

Armbruster, B. B. (2009). Note taking from lectures. In R. F. Flippo & D. C. Caverly (Eds.). *Handbook of college reading and study strategy research* (pp. 220-248). New York, NY: Lawrence Erlbaum.

Baker, L. & Lombardi, B. R. (1985). Students' lecture notes and their relation to test performance. *Teaching of Psychology, 12*, 28–32.

Burchfield, C.M. & Sapington, J. (2000). Compliance with required reading assignments. *Teaching of Psychology, 27*, 58-60.

Carney, A., Fry, S., Gabriele, R., & Ballard, M. (2008). Reeling in the big fish: Changing pedagogy to encourage the completion of reading assignments. *College Teaching, 56*(4), 195-200.

Clump, M. A., Bauer, H., & Bradley, C. (2004). The extent to which psychology students read textbooks: A multiple class analysis of reading across the psychology curriculum. *Journal of Instructional Psychology, 31*, 227-229.

Jacobs, L. F. & Hyman, J. S. (2006). *Professors' guide to getting good grades in college.* New York, NY: Harper Collins Publishers.

Kiewra, K. A., DuBois, N. F., Christian, D., & McShane, A. (1988). Providing study notes: Comparison of three types of notes for review. *Journal of Educational Psychology, 80*, 595-597.

O'Donnell, A. & Dansereau, D. F. (1993). Learning from lectures: Effects of cooperative review. *Journal of experimental education, 61*, 116-125.

Pardini, E. A., Domizi, D. P., Forbes, D. A., & Pettis, G. V. (2005). Parallel note-taking: A strategy for effective use of webnotes. *Journal of College Reading and Learning, 35*(2), 38-55.

Peverly, S., Ramaswamy, V., Brown, C., Sumowski, J., Alidoost, M., & Garner, J. (Feb, 2007). What predicts skill in lecture note-taking? *Journal of Educational Psychology, 99*(1), 167-180.

Terry, W. S. (2006). *Learning and memory* (3rd ed.). Boston: Pearson Education, Inc.

Titsworth, B. S. & Kiewra, K. A. (2004). Spoken organizational lecture cues and student note taking as facilitators of student learning. *Contemporary Educational Psychology, 29*, 447-461.

Williams, R. L. & Eggert, A. C. (2002). Note-taking in college classes: Student patterns and instructional strategies. *The Journal of General Education, 51*(3), 174-199.

Wirt, J., Choy, S., Greald, D., Provasnik, S., Rooney, P., & Watanabe, S. (2001). *The condition of education.* Washington, DC: Government Printing Office (NCES Publication No. 2001072).

Everyday learning refers to the learning that takes place outside the walls of the classroom. In other words, everyday learning is the day-to-day studying and reviewing of your class material. Aside from where and when to study, your learning preferences guide your studying. These preferences are probably a blend of several approaches. You may have a strong visual orientation, for example, and enjoy studying with others. Perhaps you are also someone who follows the phrase, "seeing is believing." This section introduces you to a variety of learning styles and preferences as well as multiple intelligences. By identifying your preferences and intelligence, you will make your study sessions more productive, which in turn will help you perform better on tests.

3.1 Where and when to study

The right place and time to study is different for different people. You may prefer to study in a quiet library, or in the comfort of your own home, or perhaps you prefer to study in a bustling coffee shop. While it is important to choose a location in which you are comfortable, you must also ask yourself whether the spot you choose is an effective study site. As such, a balance between preference and practicality must be struck when deciding where to study. A similar balance must be found when deciding when to study. Although your schedule may restrict the time of day you can study, you should try to study when you are most alert. The purpose of this section is to discuss the answers to the following two questions:

- Where is the best place to study?

- When is the best time to study?

Where is the best place to study?

Your studying will be most effective if you choose a place to study that is right for you. Research has suggested that the best place to study is the same place, or at least a place in a similar setting, that you originally learned the material (Terry, 2006). This means that if most of your learning occurs in the classroom, then the best place to study is probably a classroom. If you are unable to study in a classroom, then a library may be the next best place to study because it closely resembles the environment of a typical classroom. Wherever you choose, remember that a study spot with few distractions will help you focus better on the material (Fry, 2005).

 Hands-on strategies

The following hands-on strategies may help you stay focused in the place you choose to study.

- **Study in a place similar to where the learning first took place.** If you learned the material in a quiet setting, study in a quiet setting. If you learned the material in an interactive classroom, try to recreate that environment.

- **Use decent lighting.** Ensure that your study area has adequate lighting. This will keep you from straining while you read your material in addition to helping you stay awake and alert.

- **Study in a room with a comfortable temperature.** You do not want your study environment to be too hot or too cold. A cooler room temperature is preferable to one that is excessively warm since warm temperatures may promote sleepiness.

- **Have plenty of space.** Your study area should provide ample space for you to organize your study materials in an orderly manner. Everything you need should be easily accessible without requiring a great deal of maneuvering.

- **Avoid distractions.** Try to study in a place with few external distractions. The more focused you are during your studying, the more productive you will be.

When is the best time to study?

The best time to study is different for different people. Just as the best place to study depends on several individual preferences, the best time to study does, too. It is also dependent on your schedule. Research suggests you figure out if you are a morning, afternoon, or evening person and try to complete the bulk of your studying during this time (Terry, 2006). Moreover, if you can predict when you will be most alert, then you should try to study at this time. When you are most alert, you will be most productive (Fry, 2005; Lamonte, 2007; Leber, Turk-Browne, & Chun, 2008; Terry, 2006).

 Hands-on strategies

The following hands-on strategies may help you find the best time to study.

- **Study during your alert times.** If you are a morning person, get up early in the morning and study. If you are an evening person, make sure you are studying at night. In either case, make sure you allow yourself to get a good night's sleep.

- **Take advantage of your alert times.** If your brain is alert, then you should take advantage of that time and study. Your studying will be most effective when you are alert.

- **Rearrange other activities.** If extracurricular activities, such as jobs or athletics, take up a lot of your time, see if you can rearrange your activities so that you can study at your most alert times. Otherwise, determine which days of the week you can study at your most alert times and do so.

- **Schedule classes during your alert times.** If you have a choice, sign up for the class during the time you are most alert. This will help you retain more information and write good notes.

- **Try studying at different times of the day.** If you're not sure if you're a morning or night person, try studying at different times of the day until you find what time is best for you.

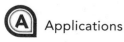 Applications

1. Think of three locations at which you enjoy studying. Go through the following checklist to determine if each location has the qualities of a good place to study. Add other items to the list that you consider important.

   ☐ Sufficient lighting
   ☐ Moderate temperature
   ☐ Ample table space
   ☐ Few distractions
   ☐ _____
   ☐ _____
   ☐ _____

2. What time of day are you most alert? What time of day are you able to do most of your studying? Are your answers to these two questions the same or different? If they are the same, can you think of ways to make your studying even more effective? If your answers to the two questions are different, list some possible options for improving the effectiveness of your study sessions.

   Possible response: Rearrange your schedule so that you can study during your most alert time. Use weekends, when possible, to study during your most alert times. If necessary, stay up later or get up earlier to capture the times you study most effectively. When selecting classes to take for the following quarter, trimester, or semester, select sections that are offered during your most alert times.

Summary

Your decision about where and when to study will affect your study sessions. You should try to select a study environment similar to the environment in which you first learned the material; however, other study areas are fine as long as distractions are kept to a minimum. In addition, try to study during the times that you are most alert. By giving careful thought to where and when you study, you may perform better on your next test.

 Review

Determine whether the following statements are true or false. Select the correct response. Answers are provided at the end of this book.

1. True   False   It is preferable to study in a warm room than in a cool room.

2. True   False   It is important to study under conditions similar to those in which you will be tested.

3. True   False   It is better to study with distractions because the real world is full of distractions.

4. True   False   It is best to study first thing in the morning.

3.2 Reading strategies

Have you ever felt overwhelmed by all the reading you are assigned in each of your classes? Some instructors may not expect you to read the assigned material word for word, but others may hold you responsible for every detail. Developing strategies for effectively reading texts is key to being successful. The purpose of this section is to answer the following question:

- What are some strategies for reading all my class material?

What are some strategies for reading all my class material?

Reading hundreds of pages of material in a week can be overwhelming. Finding strategies to help you read and process all this material is necessary. Research suggests that you try to apply or connect the new information you are reading about to prior information (Raphael & Au, 2005). When reading the material, research also suggests that you scan the material for key words and make sure you are taking good notes on the material (see section 2.2) (Peverly et al., 2007; Raphael & Au, 2005; Terry, 2006; Titsworth & Kiewra, 2004; Williams & Eggert, 2002). The more organized your approach for the reading, the more successful you will be at remembering what you have read.

 Hands-on strategies

The following hands-on strategies may help you be more successful in remembering the material you read.

- **Review the assigned text.** Before delving into the details of an assigned reading, scan through the introduction, summary, key terms and definitions, and any stated learning objectives.

- **Outline the text.** Write Roman numerals (I, II, ...) for major divisions, capital letters for minor divisions, and Arabic numerals (1, 2, ...) for further detail. You may choose to outline the text on a separate sheet of paper or write in the assigned reading. Highlighting these parts of the reading will help get you focused on the content and what to expect in the readings.

- **Underline topic sentences.** This will help you remember the important concepts when you review the text. It will also help you keep focused while you're reading.

- **Write vocabulary words, concepts, and dates in the margin.** Writing in the margins places an extra emphasis on the information. Be sure to draw an arrow from the margin to the place in the text that the word, concept, or date appears. By writing this information in the text, it is easy to review at a later time and the act of writing it will help you remember the information, too.

- **Know the expectations of the assigned readings.** Are you responsible for every detail or just the big picture? The answer to this question may be clear just by attending class and listening to the information the instructor presents.

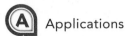

Applications

The two excerpts presented below in Figure 3.1 and Figure 3.2 are examples of how to outline, underline, and write information in the margins of an assigned reading. After reviewing these examples, try applying this technique to your next reading. The following list may help you:

- Use Roman numerals for main headings.

- Use capital letters for main subheadings.

- Use Arabic numbers for all other headings.

- Underline topic sentences.

- Write key words, definitions, and dates in the margins and draw an arrow to where they appear in the text.

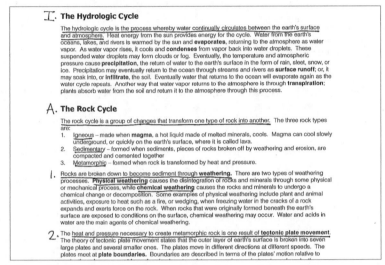

Figure 3.1 Example of outlining headings and underlining topic sentences.

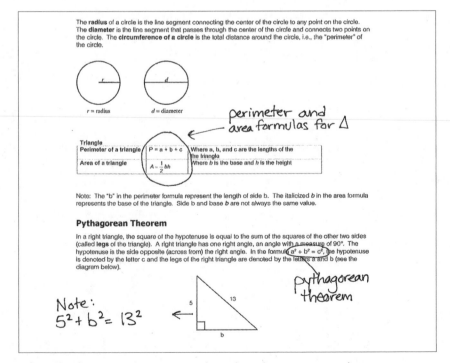

Figure 3.2. Example of writing in the margins and matching the comments to the text.

Summary

This section introduced you to techniques for reading assigned material. First, you should skim the reading and capture the main idea. Then, using some type of hands-on technique, such as underlining or outlining, read the text for more detail. Following the suggestions presented in this section takes time, but it will help you retain the information and save you time in the long run.

(R) Review

Determine whether the following statements are true or false. Select the correct response. Answers are provided at the end of this book.

1. True   False   It is a poor use of time to try to connect the material you are currently reading about in an assignment to information you have already learned.

2. True   False   The organization of your notes is related to how well you remember what you have read.

3. True   False   Highlighting and writing in a textbook makes it more difficult to remember the reading material because there is so much extra writing in the book.

3.3 Learning styles

Learning styles refer to your learning preferences. Do you prefer to learn by listening to lectures, conducting hands-on experiments, or reading textbooks? Are you someone who often asks "Why?", "What?", "How?", or "What if?" Or, would you describe yourself as someone who is always on the move and likes to relate new information to information you already know? Depending on your answer, your learning style may be defined in multiple ways. Moreover, you may be able to adapt your learning style to the type of instruction you are receiving (Vermunt & Vermetten, 2004). The purpose of this section is to help you determine your learning style(s) by discussing three learning style models and offering study strategies for each model. More specifically, this section will answer the following questions:

- How should an auditory, tactile, or visual learner study? (ATV — Model 1)

- Which one-word question do you often ask? (Kolb — Model 2)

- How do you take in and process new information? (Felder — Model 3)

How should an auditory, tactile, or visual learner study? (ATV — Model 1)

Do you know your learning style? In other words, do you know how you learn best? Is it through pictures? Sounds? Actions? The better you know yourself and how you learn best, the better you will do on tests. Research has shown that most learners fall into one of three categories: auditory, tactile (or kinesthetic), or visual learners (Terry, 2006). Auditory learners prefer to hear the information spoken. Tactile learners prefer active learning, such as conducting laboratory experiments. Visual learners prefer seeing a picture or graphic (Jensen & Nickelsen, 2008). Identifying the learning style(s) that best describes you will help you be more productive when studying.

 Hands-on strategies

The following list of hands-on strategies is organized by the different learning styles. Depending on your style (see the Application portion of this section), these strategies may help increase the effectiveness of your studying.

- **Auditory learners**
  - Review material aloud with other students.
  - Record a summary of your notes and listen to them.
  - Read notes aloud.
  - Personalize information by turning it into a song or mnemonic device.
  - Explain concepts to others.
  - Talk to the instructor.
  - Work in groups.

- **Tactile learners**
  - Create a hands-on model or display of the concepts.
  - If possible, use hands-on learning tools to help develop an understanding of the material.

- **Visual learners**
  - Use graphic organizers such as charts, outlines, and diagrams to represent content.
  - View a video of the material, if possible.
  - Read material in textbooks.
  - Read a variety of books or pamphlets on the subject.
  - Request written course objectives and study the content outline.
  - Highlight text.

Which one-word question do you often ask? (Kolb — Model 2)

Are you someone who prefers hands-on experimentation or working with abstract concepts? For example, in a math class, would you learn better if your instructor used a hands-on model to demonstrate how to solve an algebraic equation, or are you content with just seeing the teacher walk through the steps on a board? Are you someone who prefers to think about a situation for a while, or do you like to act on the knowledge that you already have? These types of questions address how you take in and process information.

Research suggests that people can be divided into four categories based on how they take in and process information (Kolb, 1981). These categories can be simply understood by figuring out what type of question you ask most often (Stice, 1987). Of the following four questions, which do you find yourself asking most often: "Why?", "What?", "What if?", or "How?" The following list describes the learners most closely associated with these types of questions (Kolb, 1981; Stice, 1987; Terry, 2006):

- "Why?" people are reflective, concrete thinkers. They tend to be imaginative, good at brainstorming ideas, interested in people, emotional, and prefer subjects in the humanities and liberal arts field.

- "What?" people are reflective, abstract thinkers. They enjoy inductive reasoning, are not terribly interested in socializing, work well with abstract ideas, but are not too interested in practical components of theories. These people tend to be interested in the research and planning fields.

- "What if?" people are active, concrete thinkers. They excel in adapting to situations and enjoy taking risks. These types of people tend to ask someone for information instead of spending time to think it through themselves; consequently, these people may come across as pushy or impatient with others. These people prefer fields that involve solving problems by trial and error.

- "How?" people are active, abstract thinkers. They prefer working with objects instead of people. These types of people enjoy studying fields such as physical science.

 ## Hands-on strategies

Depending on the type of question you tend to ask, the following hands-on strategies may give you some tips to consider the next time you study.

- "Why?" person (a.k.a. the diverger)

  o **Brainstorm different ways to think about the material.** The more connections you can make with the material, the better you will learn it.

  o **Study with people.** Because you probably work well with others, take advantage of this strength and study with peers.

  o **Take courses in the humanities and liberal arts.** Because you probably enjoy taking these types of courses, you will probably do well in them, too.

- "What?" person (a.k.a. the assimilator)

  o **Spend more time studying alone.** Your learning style lends itself well to working independently and figuring out abstract concepts on your own.

  o **Don't forget the applications of theories.** You may be inclined to understand the big picture, but don't forget to understand the practical components of a concept. You may have to apply your knowledge in the "real world" or on a test.

  o **Take courses involving research.** You may enjoy researching information and using that information to form an abstract concept. When you enroll in courses, try to make sure that research is a component of the course. You'll enjoy it more and you will do better with a more practical, application-driven course.

- "What if?" person (a.k.a. the accommodator)

  o **Use trial and error to help learn concepts.** Since you prefer to use trial and error instead of thinking though the steps of why something may or may not work, go ahead and use that method to your advantage. When a trial-and-error experiment finally works, you will probably remember how it worked.

  o **Remember to be patient.** Stay focused on the task at hand. Don't try to answer another "What if?" question before the first one is answered. Getting caught up in "What if this were to happen?" questions will lead you off task and probably get you frustrated.

- ○ **Take courses that complement a trial-and-error learning style.** You probably would benefit from probability and statistic courses and laboratory courses that would allow you to conduct several trial-and-error experiments in order to learn the desired outcome.

- "How?" person (a.k.a. the converger)

  - ○ **Build models.** The more manipulatives and models that are available for you to use, the more you will learn. Use any materials, such as boxes, strings, or cans, to model concepts you are learning in class.

  - ○ **Take courses with lab components.** Since one of your strengths is working with models and seeing how things work, you would do well in courses with lab components, such as a chemistry or engineering course.

How do you take in and process new information? (Felder — Model 3)

Do you absorb information better by using your senses (such as sight and hearing) or by thinking about information and how it relates to other information you already know? Do you prefer to learn information through pictures or by discussion? Are you an active studier (always writing or doing something with your hands or feet) or are you more reflective? Do you prefer to learn information sequentially or to be given the big picture first and then learn the details?

These questions relate directly to how you perceive, process, and understand information (Felder, 1993; Felder & Silverman, 1988). If you prefer to absorb information though your senses and rely less on intuition, then you are probably a practical type of person who likes to solve problems, is careful but slow, and tends not to be very comfortable with symbolic language. If you are more intuitive, then you are probably imaginative, do not mind variety and complex problem solving, are quick to get things done, but you may be a little careless (Felder, 1993; Felder & Silverman, 1988).

If you are someone who prefers some form of physical activity while studying, then you are probably the type of learner who learns from doing and benefits from working in groups. If you are a reflective learner, however, you probably enjoy working alone and processing information internally and without much physical activity (Felder, 1993; Felder & Silverman, 1988).

If you are someone who prefers to learn information one piece at a time in a sequential manner, then it may take time for you to get the big picture. If you are the type of learner who absorbs bits and pieces of information and tries to create a large picture with this information, you are a more global learner. Global learners tend to struggle with details at first, but once they get the big picture, they truly understand the concept (Felder, 1993; Felder & Silverman, 1988).

If you are someone who prefers to learn by seeing, then you learn best by reading materials, viewing videos, or seeing something happen. This type of learner contrasts with a verbal learner. If you are someone who prefers to learn by hearing, then you learn best by discussing topics and working with other people.

 Hands-on strategies

The following hands-on strategies offer suggestions for ways to improve your studying based on your learning preference. The strategies are organized according to Felder's model.

- Sensory learners (use your five senses)

  - ○ **Relate information to the real world.** You will probably remember information better if you can find some type of real-world context for the new information.

  - ○ **Ask for examples or diagrams.** Because you learn best through your senses, ask for examples, diagrams, or models during lectures.

  - ○ **Create your own examples or diagrams.** Because you are a more concrete learner, creating examples and diagrams or models of the information will help you remember the information.

- Intuitive learners (use your intuition)

  - ○ **Link information into one concept.** The more information that you can tie together into one concept, the easier it will be for you to remember it.

  - ○ **Read carefully.** Don't be in a rush to get through an assignment or test. Take the time to read and complete the assignment carefully and thoroughly.

    o **Check your work.** Because you rely on your intuition, you may skip the important step of checking your work on an assignment or test. Make sure you are taking the time to check your work. This will help you avoid making careless mistakes.

- Active learners (learn from doing)

    o **Put your learning to use.** Find a hands-on way to apply the information you have learned.

    o **Take advantage of lab classes.** You probably enjoy and learn best in courses with a lab component.

    o **Work with others.** Review and discuss ideas with others. The more active you are in the learning process, the better you'll remember the information.

- Reflective learners (learn from thinking it through)

    o **Read material at least twice.** Because you need time to think about the material to understand it, take the time to read through the material more than once. This will help your thoughts become clearer as you absorb more details.

    o **Give yourself time to reflect.** Don't approach an assignment with the goal of just getting it done; spend time with the material so you have time to think about it and truly understand it.

    o **Rewrite your notes or take notes as you study.** When you write, you tend to think more about the material. Because you are a reflective learner, spending the time rewriting notes or taking notes as you study will help you remember the information.

- Sequential learner (learn in steps)

    o **Have a series of steps to follow to learn the material.** Because you work best in a sequential manner, make sure you have a series of steps to take to master the material. For example,

       ■ Step 1. Scan the chapter headings.

       ■ Step 2. Skim the chapter for main ideas.

       ■ Step 3. Read the chapter once.

       ■ Step 4. Reread the chapter for more detail.

    o **Keep your notes in a logical order.** Be sure to date your notes and keep them in an order that makes sense when you go back to read it. If your notes are not sequential, rewrite them or outline them into an order that makes sense to you.

    o **Know steps in a process.** If a problem requires a series of steps to follow, such as a math problem, make sure you know them.

    o **Don't forget the big picture.** Make sure you understand the big picture of what you're learning. Know how the steps you've learned fit into this picture.

- Global learner (learn by the big picture)

    o **Ask for the big picture.** Don't be shy to ask your instructor for the big picture so that you don't get lost in the details.

    o **Look for the details that support the big picture.** Once you have the big picture, make sure you spend the time to fill in the details.

    o **Take time to figure out the big picture.** Because you learn best by having the big picture, make sure you study the details of your notes or text and pull out the main concepts.

    o **Preview reading assignments.** Before reading an assignment in detail, make sure you get the big picture of your assigned reading by previewing any major headings and skimming the material for the general idea. Once you have the big picture, then read the assigned material for more detail.

- Visual learner (learn by seeing)

    o Refer to the hands-on strategies for an visual learner in the "How should an auditory, tactile, or visual learner study" section of this chapter.

- Verbal learners (learn by talking)

    o Refer to the hands-on strategies for an auditory learner in the "How should an auditory, tactile, or visual learner study" section of this chapter.

Applications

1. Do you think you are an auditory, visual, or tactile learner? Do an Internet search for "Learning styles inventory" + Auditory + Visual + Tactile. Complete at least two inventories to determine if you are an auditory, visual, or kinesthetic (tactile) learner. Are the results of the two surveys the same or different? Do the results of the surveys surprise you? Did you learn anything about yourself from the surveys? Consider the results of these surveys and your own intuition about your learning preference. Apply some of the hands-on strategies suggested in this section the next time you sit down to study.

2. What type of learner do you think best describes your learning style using Kolb's model? Are you a reflective thinker or active? Do you learn concrete or abstract concepts easier? Perform an Internet search for "Learning styles inventory" + Kolb. Complete at least two inventories to help you determine which type of learner you are based on Kolb's model. Then, refer to the hands-on strategies provided in this chapter to see if any of the strategies may help you improve your next study session.

3. Are you a sensory or an intuitive learner? Are you an active or reflective learner? Are you a sequential or global learner? Search the Internet for "Learning styles inventory" + Felder. Complete at least two inventories. Based on the results, what strategies should you implement when studying to ensure that you are benefiting the most from your study sessions? Can you think of other strategies that may also help you?

Summary

The purpose of this section was to introduce you to three learning style models. The first model may help you determine if you are more an auditory, tactile, or visual learner. The second model may help you determine if you are more a "Why?", "What?", "What if?", or "How?" learner. The third model may help you determine how you take in and process new information. The applications portion of this section provided a way to help you figure out your learning style strengths. The hands-on strategies then directed you to ways to capitalize on your learning strengths in order to be more successful in the classroom and on tests.

Ⓡ Review

Determine whether statements 1 to 4 are true or false. Select the correct response. Choose the best option for questions 5 and 6. The answers are provided at the end of this book.

1. True   False   Auditory learners will benefit most from graphic organizers.

2. True   False   Visual learners often prefer to learn from a textbook.

3. True   False   Kolb's model categorizes learners based on how they take in and process information.

4. True   False   Kolb's model divides people into either reflective or active learners.

5. Which of the following hands-on strategies are most appropriate for an intuitive learner?

     A. Checking your work
     B. Following a set of steps to complete a problem
     C. Working in study groups
     D. Concentrating on grasping the big picture

6. Which of the following hands-on strategies are most appropriate for a reflective learner?

     A. Watching a DVD of the material
     B. Finding a hands-on way to apply the material
     C. Taking time to think about your notes
     D. Organizing your notes in a logical sequence

3.4 Multiple intelligences

Multiple intelligences refer to your intellectual strengths. These strengths are different than your learning style preference, because your strengths are not the same as your preferences. Stated another way, your learning style is influenced by your multiple intelligences. The purpose of this section is to answer and provide strategies related to the following question:

- What are your multiple intelligences?

What are your multiple intelligences?

Have you ever heard the phrase "multiple intelligences?" Howard Gardner, the researcher responsible for developing and coining this phrase, defined multiple intelligences as "the human ability to solve problems" (Checkley, 1997). For example, are you musically inclined? Are you able to have conversations with just about anyone? If you answered "yes" to the music question, then perhaps you have musical intelligence. If you answered "yes" to the conversation question, then perhaps you have interpersonal (or social) intelligence. (Checkley, 1997; Moran, Kornhaber, & Gardner, 2006). The more you know about your own knowledge and intelligences, the better you will be able to use these strengths while studying and learning.

There are many types of intelligences. The following list describes some of these intelligences. As you read though the list, think about which type of intelligence describes you. A detailed description of these intelligences can be found in Howard Gardner's (1983) *Frames of mind: Theory of multiple intelligences*. The descriptions in the following list are suggested by Checkley (1997), Jensen and Nickelsen (2008), and Moran, Kornhaber, and Gardner (2006).

- **Bodily/Kinesthetic Intelligence** (Physical learner) — These types of learners learn best by doing. In other words, they learn best by working with concrete or hands-on models instead of learning by more abstract methods, such as listening to a lecture.

- **Intrapersonal Intelligence** (Solitary learner) — These types of learners know themselves well; i.e., they know what they can and cannot do. These types of learners tend to spend time thinking and reflecting on information.

- **Interpersonal Intelligence** (Social learner) — These types of learners enjoy others. They communicate well and learn well with other people.

- **Logical/Mathematical Intelligence** (Logical learner) — These types of learners enjoy working with cause and effect relationships and working with numbers.

- **Musical/Rhythmic Intelligence** (Rhythmic learner) — These types of learners are good at remembering patterns and rhythms.

- **Verbal/Linguistic Intelligence** (Verbal learner) — These types of learners use language to express themselves, such as through poetry or oral prose.

- **Visual/Spatial Intelligence** (Visual learner) — These types of learners visualize three-dimensional objects well and also prefer to write out information into an organized fashion, such as an outline or diagram.

- **Auditory Intelligence** (Aural learner) — These types of learners learn through listening and tend to be easily distracted by outside noises. These types of learners also tend to be quite chatty.

- **Naturalist Intelligence** (Natural learner) — These types of learners can tell the difference between items in the world, such as the differences between plant species or different types of animals or rock formations.

Hands-on strategies

The following list of hands-on strategies is organized by the different types of intelligences. Once you have identified your intelligences, these strategies may help you use them to increase your next test score.

- Bodily/Kinesthetic Intelligence

  ○ Create diagrams of your notes.

  ○ Model concepts.

  ○ Play a game of charades with your friends in the class to help study.

- Intrapersonal Intelligence
  - Primarily study alone.
  - Minimize group work because it may be distracting to you.
- Interpersonal Intelligence
  - Study in groups.
  - Try to teach someone the information on which you will be tested.
- Logical/Mathematical Intelligence
  - Try to identify a problem and then identify what caused the problem and the effects of that problem.
  - Try to reason through difficult concepts and understand the logic behind the idea.
- Musical/Rhythmic Intelligence
  - Write information you're studying into a song.
  - Play background music while you're studying.
- Verbal/Linguistic Intelligence
  - Rewrite the information you are studying into a story or poem.
  - Pretend you are teaching someone this concept via an e-mail or letter.
  - If given the option, choose to give oral presentations instead of written presentations.
- Visual/Spatial Intelligence
  - Diagram your notes.
  - Picture real-life objects or events related to the topic of study.
- Auditory Intelligence
  - Record your lectures and listen to the recording.
  - Attend the same lecture at two different times (if the instructor teaches the same course twice).
- Naturalist Intelligence
  - Relate as much information as you can to nature.
  - Identify the similarities and differences between concepts.

 Application

Search the Internet for "multiple intelligence inventory." Complete at least two inventories to help you determine your multiple intelligences. How does knowing this information help you?

Summary

The section has introduced you to the many types of multiple intelligences first introduced by Howard Gardner. By completing the application part of this section, you may have a better idea of the intelligences that define you. Applying strategies that complement your intelligences may help you improve the productivity of your next study session.

 Review

Choose the best option for the three questions below. Answers are provided at the end of this book.

1. Which of the following multiple intelligences best describes an artist?

    A. Kinesthetic intelligence
    B. Rhythmic intelligence
    C. Visual intelligence
    D. Auditory intelligence

2. Which of the following multiple intelligences best describes a statistician?

    A. Interpersonal intelligence
    B. Verbal intelligence
    C. Logical intelligence
    D. Naturalist intelligence

3. Which of the following multiple intelligences best describes an athlete?

    A. Kinesthetic intelligence
    B. Intrapersonal intelligence
    C. Rhythmic intelligence
    D. Verbal intelligence

3.5 Tips for remembering facts

Every class you take will require you to learn information. Some of that information will be easy for you to learn and remember; other information will be more difficult to retain. Sometimes, less challenging material is the most difficult to remember. For example, definitions, dates, and formulas are basic facts and are not challenging on the face of it. These facts, however, can be a burden to remember. The purpose of this section is to answer the following question:

- What are some tips for remembering facts?

What are some tips for remembering facts?

Have you ever been in a class that requires a lot of memorization, such as a foreign language class? Unless you have one or more strategies for tackling all of the memorization, the amount of material you have to learn may seem overwhelming. No matter what type of class you take, you will encounter facts or vocabulary words that you will have to store in your memory and be able to recall (McClanahan, 2009).

Research offers several methods for studying and remembering factual information. One such method involves using mnemonic devices to help you learn vocabulary definitions or lists of words (Stalder, 2005; Terry, 2006). The acronym "HOMES," for example, is a mnemonic device used to help remember names of the five great lakes: Huron, Ontario, Michigan, Erie, and Superior. Memory techniques like this create triggers in your mind to help you remember the information when it is needed (Levin, 1986). The purpose of this section is to provide you with some hands-on strategies for remembering formulas and definitions.

 ## Hands-on strategies

The following list of hands-on strategies may help you memorize facts.

- **Look for patterns in the fact.** Patterns are easier to remember than facts without patterns.

- **Develop sayings for facts.** Create your own method for remembering a fact. For example, if you are trying to remember how to spell "desert" and "dessert," perhaps the saying "You are alone in a desert, but you eat dessert with people" would help you remember that "desert" has one "s" while "dessert" has two.

- **Group related facts together.** It's easier to memorize facts that are related to each other than facts that are not related.

- **Write a story or use rhymes to help remember facts.** Develop a story with seemingly unrelated facts. If you can make the facts seem related, you may remember them better. If you can make the story rhyme, it will even be more memorable.

- **Practice using the fact.** The best way to learn formulae "inside out" is to practice using them.

- **Make flash cards.** Write the term or formula on one side and the definition or calculation on the other. Review the cards a few times a day. When you have learned the information, save the cards for review at exam time.

- **Fold a piece of paper in half and write the fact on one side and answers on the other side.** This is similar to flashcards, except you can see more than one word or formula at a time.

- **Speak the fact.** The more of your five senses that you can involve in the studying, the better chance you have of remembering it.

- **Explain the fact to a peer.** Teaching is one of the best ways to learn.

- **Remember common acronyms or phrases.** Common sayings are common for a reason — they help people remember. For example, the acronym "PEMDAS" and the phrase "Please Excuse My Dear Aunt Sally" are common memory devices taught in math classes to help students remember the order of operations (Parentheses first, then Exponents, Multiplication, Division, Addition, Subtraction).

- **Develop your own acronym or phrase.** If there is a list of facts associated with a concept, write out the facts and try to create a saying using the first letters of each word.

- **Write a song using the facts.** This may sound silly, but if you can put the facts to music, you may remember it better.

- **Create visual images.** Try to create a pleasant picture that your mind can go to and associate with a fact, such as a daisy for a character named Daisy or a heart for Valentine's Day.

- **Look at the word itself for memory cues.** A fact may have some mnemonic device within itself. For example, "Mr. Abraham Lincoln" contains 16 letters and Lincoln was the 16th president of the United States.

- **Write the fact out several times a day.** You will probably learn the material if you repeat it to yourself enough times. Writing out a definition several times a day for several days will help get the information into your memory.

- **Use previous knowledge.** Is there part of the word or fact that you already know? If you can apply previous knowledge to the new fact, you'll remember it better and quicker. For example, the word "biostatistics" may be new to you, but if you know that "bio" refers to life, then you can probably figure out that this word means "statistics related to life."

 Applications

1. Consider the following sets of commonly misspelled words. What are some mnemonic devices that you could create to help remember when to use each word in the set?

   principal (noun)
   principle (noun)

   then
   than

   lead (noun)
   led (verb)

   Possible response: The word "pal" is in "principal." This may help you remember that a "principal" is a person. "Principle" means a foundational concept.

   "Then" rhymes with "when," which may help you remember that it is used to describe the next step or used in an if-then statement. "Than" is used in comparisons.

   The word "led" is short, while "lead" is a little heavier. This may help you remember that the past tense of "to lead" is "led", while "lead" refers to the heavy metal.

2. Study the following list of words for 30 seconds. Then, cover the list and try to write down as many words as you can remember in the space provided.

   dog
   alligator
   grass
   rain
   bone
   lettuce
   ice

   _____
   _____
   _____
   _____
   _____
   _____
   _____

Now, group the words into categories, such as by color or alphabetical order or any other way that makes sense to you, and write them in the space provided.

———————————————————
———————————————————
———————————————————
———————————————————
———————————————————
———————————————————

Study the list for 20 seconds. Cover up the list and try to write down all the words you can remember in the space provided.

———————————————————
———————————————————
———————————————————
———————————————————
———————————————————
———————————————————
———————————————————

Did your recall improve? It should have improved because you devised a technique for reducing seven seemingly unrelated words into groups of related words. Now, try this technique with lists of facts you are trying to memorize for one of your classes. Just thinking about the words and how they go together will help you remember the facts.

3. Consider the following list of words:

   lotion
   globe
   cat
   red
   water
   kiwi
   monitor
   carpet

Study this list of words for 45 seconds and concentrate on remembering the words in the order they appear. Now, cover this list and try to write down as many words in order that you can in the space provided:

———————————————————
———————————————————
———————————————————
———————————————————
———————————————————
———————————————————
———————————————————
———————————————————

Now, look back at the list of 8 words. Take 2 minutes to create a story with these words beginning with "lotion" and ending with "carpet." After these 2 minutes are up, cover up the list and try to write down the list of words in order. Use the space provided.

———————————————————
———————————————————
———————————————————
———————————————————
———————————————————
———————————————————
———————————————————
———————————————————

Did your recall improve? Hopefully, by creating a story involving all of the words, you were able to remember them better. Try using this technique with the next list of chronological events that you are asked to learn.

4. One of the best ways to remember facts is to practice, practice, practice. If you find that you simply cannot remember a list of facts, go through this list and see if there's a strategy you haven't tried yet. You may be surprised to find that a new strategy works.

- Make flash cards

- Fold a piece of paper in half and write the fact on one side and answers on the other side (The example below could be used to memorize the first 13 states to join the Union and when they joined. The left side lists the states and the right side lists the years. Fold the paper in half to form a study sheet.)

DE, PE, NJ	1787
GA, CT, MA, MD, SC, NH, VA, NY	1788
NC	1789
RI	1790

- Say the facts aloud

- Explain the facts to a friend

- Create or use common acronyms or phrases to help you remember the facts

- Write a song using the facts

- Create visual images

- Examine each fact separately and look for cues within the fact to help you remember it

- Practice the facts by any of the above methods several times a day and for multiple days

- Use your current knowledge to help you learn the new facts

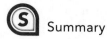 Summary

Although the amount of information you have to learn at any one time may seem overwhelming or even impossible at times, consider some of the tips suggested in this section to help ease that anxiety. The mnemonic devices and study strategies presented in this section may not only help you remember the facts, but it may make your studying a little more enjoyable — especially if you can come up with some memory tricks with your friends.

R Review

Decide if the following two statements are true or false. Then, answer question 3. The answers are provided at the end of this book.

1. True   False   Mnemonic devices can help with memorization.

2. True   False   It is best to try and memorize a list of terms in one session as opposed to over multiple days.

3. Consider the following sets of words and definitions. Create a mnemonic device for each set that could help someone remember when to use each word.

         A. naval: relating to ships and the sea
            navel: bellybutton
         B. over do: to do in excess
            overdue: past date of payment
         C. roll: to move by revolving or turning around and around
            role: a part in a play

References

Checkley, K. (1997). *The first seven . . . and the eighth: A conversation with Howard Gardner.* Retrieved April 20, 2009 from http://www.nnrec.org/profdev/plt/handouts/FirstSevenAndEighth.pdf

Felder, R. M. (1993). Reaching the second tier: Learning and teaching styles in college science education. *Journal of College Science Teaching, 22*(5), 286-290.

Felder, R. M. and L. K. Silverman (1988). Learning and teaching styles in engineering education. *Engineering education, 78*(7), 674-81.

Fry, R. (2005). *How to study.* (6th ed.). Clifton Park, NY: Delmar Learning.

Gardner, H. (1983). *Frames of mind: Theory of multiple intelligences.* New York: Basic Books.

Jensen, E. & Nickelsen, L. (2008). *Deeper learning: 7 powerful strategies for in-depth and longer-lasting learning.* Thousand Oaks, CA: Corwin Press.

Kolb, D. A. (1981). Learning styles and interdisciplinary differences. In A. Chickering (Ed.), *The modern American college* (pp. 232-255). San Francisco, CA: Jossey-Bass, Inc.

Lamonte, M. K. (2007). Test-taking strategies for CNOR certification. *Association of Perioperative Registered Nurses, 85*(2), 315-332.

Leber, A., Turk-Browne, N., & Chun, M. M. (2008). Neural predictors of moment-to-moment fluctuations in cognitive flexibility. *Proceedings of the National Academy of Sciences of the United States of America, 105*(36), 13592-13597.

Levin, J. R. (1986). Four cognitive principles of learning-strategy instruction. *Educational Psychologist, 21*, 3–17.

McClanahan, B. (2009). Help! I have kids who can't read in my world history class. *Preventing School Failure, 53*(2), 105-111.

Moran, Kornhaber, & Gardner, H. (2006). Orchestrating multiple intelligences. *Educational Leadership, 64*(1), 22-27.

Peverly, S., V. Ramaswamy, C. Brown, J. Sumowski, M. Alidoost, & J. Garner. (Feb, 2007). What predicts skill in lecture note taking? *Journal of Educational Psychology, 99*(1), 167-180.

Raphael, T. E. & Au, K. H. (2005). QAR: Enhancing comprehension and test taking across grades and content areas. *The Reading Teacher, 59*(3), 206-221.

Stalder, D. (2005). Learning and motivational benefits of acronym use in introductory psychology. *Teaching of Psychology, 32*(4), 222-228.

Stice, J. E. (1987). Using Kolb's learning cycle to improve student learning. *Engineering Education, 77*(5), 291-296.

Terry, W. S. (2006). *Learning and memory* (3rd Ed.) Boston: Pearson Education, Inc.

Titsworth, B. S. & Kiewra, K. A. (2004). Spoken organizational lecture cues and student note taking as facilitators of student learning. *Contemporary Educational Psychology, 29*, 447-461.

Vermunt, J. D. & Vermetten, Y. J. (2004). Patterns in student learning: Relationships between learning strategies, conceptions of learning, and learning orientations. *Educational Psychology Review, 16*(4), 359-384.

Williams, R. L. & Eggert, A. C. (2002). Note taking in college classes: Student patterns and instructional strategies. *The Journal of General Education, 51*(3), 174-199.

Assessments are a part of every learning experience. There are formal and informal classroom assessments, as well as more large-scale standardized assessments. The purpose of this chapter is to introduce you to and offer strategies for taking both types of assessments.

4.1 Classroom assessments

Do you ever ask yourself, "Why do I have to take so many tests?" or "What is the point of taking all of these tests?" Classroom tests provide you and your instructors with information about how you are doing in class. Assessments may take several forms, including pop quizzes, written papers, and final exams. Because assessments make up most, if not all, of your class grade, it is important to learn how to take these assessments. The purpose of this section is to answer the following question:

- What are some general strategies for taking a classroom test?

What are some general strategies for taking a classroom test?

Tests that you take for a class are designed to assess your current knowledge level, including your strengths and weaknesses. Classroom tests help inform you and your teachers about the level of mastery you have achieved on the material. Classroom tests also let the teacher know which areas you or other students are struggling with and areas that may need to be retaught (Shepard, 2006; Wolf, 2007).

Classroom assessments, in general, are well suited for measuring students' progress toward course objectives. They typically use a wide variety of formats such as true-false, short answer, essay, and multiple-choice questions. You may occasionally hear your teacher refer to a quiz as a formative test, while a final exam may be called a summative test (Shepard, 2006).

 Hands-on strategies

The following list of hands-on strategies may help you prepare to take a classroom assessment.

- **Know who wrote the test.** Did your instructor write the test for your class only, or is the test being used by several instructors? If the test were written by your instructor for your class only, you may study differently than if the test were written for several classes.

- **Know the format of the test.** Is it multiple-choice, essay, or fill-in-the-blank? You may change the way you study for a test if you know the format ahead of time.

- **Know the objectives being assessed.** On a classroom assessment, you may have a syllabus that tells you exactly the content to study. If not, ask the instructor.

- **Ask questions during the test.** On a classroom assessment, most instructors don't mind if you ask a question about the test. They may be able to help guide you in the right direction.

- **Know how you will be scored.** Will your final grade be based on how many questions you answered correctly, or will it be based on how you did in comparison to other students? This may or may not affect how you study, but it is good information to know.

- **Know how much weight will be assigned to the assessment.** Is the assessment worth 1% or 50% of your final class grade?

Application

You and a friend are taking a final exam for a Shakespeare literature class. You each took the same class, but you had different instructors. Your friend's instructor spent three weeks on *Romeo and Juliet*, while your instructor only spent one week. Your friend's instructor always gave multiple-choice exams, while your instructor only gave essay exams. You just found out that although you and your friend had different instructors, you will both be taking the same final exam. What types of questions will you want answered before taking the final exam?

> Possible response: Who is grading the final? Since each instructor had a different emphasis on the assigned readings (at least for *Romeo and Juliet*), it would be helpful to know if your instructor is grading your paper. Your instructor will know what was discussed in class and how in-depth she expects your knowledge to be of the novel. Other graders may not be privy to this information.
>
> What is the format? Since your friend's class is used to multiple-choice question tests and your class is used to essay tests, it would be helpful to know the format of the final. If it's in a different format than you are used to, you may have to practice a different set of test-taking skills before taking the final.
>
> Are you being compared to others for your final grade or is your grade just based on your responses? Will your instructor give everyone in the class an "A" if they all deserve it, or will your instructor give you a grade based on your performance as compared to others? If your final grade is based on the performance of other students, you may want to know if you will be compared only to your class or to both yours and your friend's and possibly other classes.
>
> Can you ask questions during the exam? You can ask a question, but you may not get the answer you want. However, if you don't understand the directions or are unsure on what a question is asking, you should ask the instructor.
>
> What percent of your final grade is based on the final exam? This is a fair question and should be known. If the final is only worth 5% of your grade, you may spend less time studying for it than if it were worth more—especially if you have a final exam in another class around the same time that is worth 50% of your grade.

 Summary

Testing is a natural part of education. The more familiar you are with the assessment process, the more prepared you will be to meet your educational goals. Testing provides information about your academic progress. Classroom assessments measure your current knowledge level and help your instructors make educational decisions. It is to your advantage to find out as much as possible about a classroom assessment before you actually take it. The more you know, the better you will perform.

 Review

For questions 1 to 3, determine whether each statement is true or false. Select the correct response. Answer question 4. Answers are provided at the end of this book.

1. True   False   Classroom assessments can be referred to as formative or summative.

2. True   False   Classroom assessments provide information about how you are performing nationally in a specific content area.

3. True   False   Classroom assessments may include a wide variety of question types, such as true-false, short answer, performance tasks, and multiple-choice test questions.

4. List some information you should know about a classroom assessment before taking it.

4.2 Standardized assessments

You have probably heard of the ACT®, SAT®, GRE®, ASSET®, or TOEFL®. These are just a few examples of standardized tests. When you take a standardized test, your score is being compared to other students' scores. If you took a state assessment in high school, for example, your scores on that standardized assessment were compared to other students' scores statewide. If you took or plan to take any of the tests listed above, your score will be compared to other students' scores nationwide.

Although taking standardized tests is probably not on your list of favorite things to do, you will probably have to take more of these tests at some point in your educational career. For that reason, it is worthwhile to spend time learning some general strategies for taking these types of tests. The strategies provided in this section may help you score well when you take your next standardized test. The purpose of this section is to answer the following question:

- What are some general strategies for taking a standardized test?

What are some general strategies for taking a standardized test?

At some point in your academic career, you will probably take a standardized test. There are two general types of standardized tests. One type is called a norm-referenced test. These are tests in which your score is compared to the score of other people who took the same test (Wolf, 2007). The other type is called a criterion-referenced test. These are tests in which your score reflects how well you learned a stated set of objectives. On these types of tests, your score is not compared to how others did (Haertel, 2006). Regardless of whether you are studying for a norm-referenced or criterion-referenced test, it is to your benefit to take the time to learn some general strategies for taking standardized tests.

 Hands-on strategies

The following list of hands-on strategies may help prepare you to take a standardized assessment.

- **Know the format of the test.** Is it all multiple-choice or are there other question formats? Be prepared for the item formats.

- **Know the objectives being assessed.** The objectives for a standardized test may be available through your school, a test review center, or even the companies producing the assessment (check their Web site or call them). Knowing these objectives will help guide your studying.

- **Read the directions.** Plain and simple — be sure you understand the directions.

- **Know how you are being scored.** Will you lose points for providing a wrong answer or is there no penalty for guessing?

- **If there's no penalty for guessing, guess.** If you don't lose points for guessing, then do not turn in a test with unanswered questions.

- **Familiarize yourself with strategies for completing multiple-choice and essay tests.** Refer to Chapter 6 for hands-on strategies for taking multiple-choice and essay tests.

Applications

1. There are a wide variety of question formats for a test. The following list includes some of the most common ones. Read through this list. Are there other types of question formats you've encountered? What are some strategies that you have used to answer each of these types of questions? Do you study differently for tests if you know some of these types of questions will be asked and others won't (for example, the test has multiple-choice, but no essay questions)?

- Multiple-choice

- Fill-in-the-blank

- Matching

- Short answer

- Essay

- Computation (such as for a math test)

2. The following objectives were printed as part of a standardized test:

> Students should be able to:
> • apply subject-verb agreement rules.
> • apply pronoun-antecedent agreement rules.
> • identify and use different parts of speech (e.g., possessives, pronouns, adjectives, adverbs, verbs).

Based on these objectives, it is clear that the test may include questions related to subject-verb agreement rules, and pronoun-antecedent agreement rules, and that there may be some questions requiring you to identify different parts of speech.

Now, look at the list of objectives from a standardized test that you will be taking. If you don't have such a list, try to obtain one. Otherwise, look at the list of objectives given on your class syllabus. What types of questions do you need to be prepared to answer?

3. A standardized test gives the following directions:

> The following test contains 40 multiple-choice questions. For each question you answer correctly, you will earn 1 point. For each question you answer incorrectly, you will lose ¼ of a point. For each question you omit, you will neither gain nor lose points.

A. Why is it important to read these directions?
B. How is this test being scored?
C. Should you guess on this test?

Possible response: A. These directions tell you how many questions are on the test, the type of questions on the test (multiple-choice), and the scoring directions. The testing company took the time and space to put these directions on the test because they are important for you to know.

B. You receive one point for answering the question. If you answer a question incorrectly, you lose a quarter of a point. If you don't answer the question at all, you neither gain nor lose points for that question.

C. That's up to you. If you can eliminate some of the options, you give yourself a better chance of guessing the right one.

Summary

The strategies for preparing for and taking standardized tests are similar to those for classroom assessments. Preparing for standardized tests, however, may take a little more effort on your part to get a copy of the test objectives. In addition, standardized tests tend to rely more heavily on multiple-choice questions than do classroom tests. For this reason, it's important to study strategies for answering these types of questions (see Chapter 6). In addition, because you don't take standardized tests as often as classroom tests, you are probably less familiar with the directions. Be sure to read the directions carefully on standardized tests so that you know how to answer each question and you know how you are being scored.

 Review

Determine whether the following statements are true or false. Select the correct response. Answers are provided at the end of this book.

1. True   False   The ACT® is an example of a standardized achievement test.

2. True   False   Standardized tests provide information related to student mastery of specific course outcomes.

3. True   False   Standardized tests provide detailed information about how students are performing at the national level.

4.3 Comparing classroom and standardized assessments

The goal of both classroom and standardized assessments is to find out your academic strengths and weaknesses. Classroom assessments tend to compare your knowledge to other students in your class. Standardized assessments compare your knowledge to a much larger group of students. Classroom assessments can be easily revised by your teacher to adapt to changes in course content, while standardized assessments cannot be changed since they are given to a large group of students and are often written by testing companies. Classroom assessments can often be completed within a class period and they also have a greater variety of question formats. Standardized tests may take three or more hours to complete and are often multiple-choice. Knowing how standardized tests and classroom tests are similar and different may help you understand why there are different strategies for studying and taking these assessments. The purpose of this section is to answer the question:

- How are standardized assessments similar to and different from classroom assessments?

How are standardized assessments similar to and different from classroom assessments?

Although standardized and classroom tests are similar in that they both assess your academic strengths and weaknesses, these two types of assessments are quite different. For example, standardized tests differ from classroom tests in the way they are developed, administered, and scored (Linn, 2000). Standardized tests are often developed by testing companies, are administered formally with directions that are read aloud to you and other students, and are scored by the testing company. Classroom assessments are usually written by your instructor, administered in the classroom, and these types of tests are normally scored by your instructor (Ferrara & DeMauro, 2006; Shepard, 2006). These and other differences are highlighted in Table 4.1. Becoming knowledgeable about these differences and being comfortable with some hands-on strategies that apply to both types of tests may improve your next test score.

	CLASSROOM ASSESSMENTS (SHEPARD, 2006)	STANDARDIZED ASSESSMENTS (FERRARA & DEMAURO, 2006)
Purpose	• Results are interpretable only within the classroom • Formative (e.g., teacher feedback from test) or summative (e.g., test score) • Focus of the test can also include emphasizing concepts and providing instruction	• Results are interpretable beyond the classroom (e.g., national percentile ranks, national criterion-referenced standards) • Formative (e.g., topics to study) or summative (e.g., test score) • Focus of the test is on differentiating between students of differing knowledge/ability levels
Test Specifications	• More informal, based on instruction and availability of items	• Formal, used to guide item writing • Established through a formal process (e.g., job analysis)
Development Process	• Often written entirely by the instructor	• Multiple content, editorial, and psychometric staff involved in development
Data Analysis and Scoring	• Often scored by hand • Items reviewed primarily for student performance or to gauge effectiveness of specific instruction	• Automated scoring on most, if not all, questions • Results are statistically analyzed for proper item performance and correct keys
Administration	• Conditions for administration may vary for different test takers and testing occasions	• Given under specified conditions that are consistent across administrations

Table 4.1 A Comparison of Classroom and Standardized Assessments

 Hands-on strategies

The following list suggests some hands-on strategies that can be applied to both classroom and standardized tests. These strategies may help improve your next test grade. (Note: Some of the strategies listed here have already been mentioned in this chapter, but are re-emphasized here because they apply to both types of assessments.)

- **Have a performance goal in mind.** Are you trying to achieve 80% on a classroom test or a 25 on the ACT®? Know your goal.

- **Know how much time you have to take the assessment.** In order to plan how much time you will spend on each question, you have to know how much time you have to take the entire assessment.

- **Know the format of the assessment.** Is the test multiple-choice, fill-in-the-blank, or essay?

- **Know the objectives being assessed.** Obtain a list of the objectives and study them.

- **Read the directions.** Plain and simple — be sure you understand the directions.

- **Know how much each question is worth.** Spend more time on questions that are worth more points.

- **Know how your grade is determined.** Will your final score reflect on how you did compared to others or how well you mastered the material?

 Application

As you prepare for your next test, complete the worksheet below. Answering these questions will help you get organized and prepare your mind for the test.

Preparing for a Test

What is my performance goal? _____

How much time do I have to complete the test? _____

What is the format of the test? (Select all that apply.)

    ☐ Multiple-choice

    ☐ Essay

    ☐ Fill-in-the-blank

    ☐ Short answer

    ☐ Matching

    ☐ True/False

    ☐ Other: _____

Do I have a copy of the objectives covered on the test?

    ☐ Yes

    ☐ No

What do I know about the directions (such as scoring or the number of questions)?

_____

_____

Will each question be worth the same number of points?

    ☐ Yes

    ☐ No

If no, how much will each question be worth?

_____

_____

How is your final grade on the assessment determined?

    ☐ Based on how well you mastered the material (the set of objectives)

    ☐ Based on how well you did compare to others

Summary

Although classroom and standardized tests both are designed to determine your academic strengths and weaknesses, there are several differences between the two types of tests. First, the content on the test is different. For a classroom test, your instructor most likely decided the content. This is not the case for standardized tests. Classroom tests tend to have a greater variety of question formats, while standardized tests are commonly multiple-choice. The procedures for administering and scoring, as well as for interpreting the scores are also different for the two types of assessments. Knowing the differences between the two tests and strategies for taking both tests may improve your performance on the next test you take.

 Review

Answer the following questions. Answers are provided at the end of this book.

1. Which of the following is a characteristic of most, if not all, standardized tests?

      A. Test results are often hand-scored.

      B. Test specifications are developed through a formal process.

      C. Test questions include those written by the instructor.

      D. Test results compare a student's performance to other students in the same class.

2. List 3 important pieces of information that you should know about either a standardized or classroom test before the day of the test.

References

Ferrara, S. & DeMauro, G. E. (2006). Standardized assessment of individual achievement in K-12. In R. L. Brennan (Ed.), *Educational measurement* (pp. 579-622). Westport, CT: Praeger Publishers.

Haertel, E. H. (2006). Reliability. In R. L. Brennan (Ed.), *Educational measurement* (pp. 65-110). Westport, CT: Praeger Publishers.

Linn, R. L. (2000). Assessments and accountability. *Educational Researcher, 29* (2), 4-16.

Shepard, L. A. (2006). Classroom assessment. In R. L. Brennan (Ed.), *Educational measurement* (pp. 623-646). Westport, CT: Praeger Publishers.

Wolf, P. J. (2007). Academic improvement through regular assessment. *Peabody Journal of Education, 82* (4), 690-702.

Before taking any test, there is information you should know. For example, you should know the format and purpose of the test. You should have a plan for preparing for the test and you should know what you can do during the days leading up to the test that can help lead to successful performance on the test.

5.1 Format and purpose of a test

The format and purpose of a test are two characteristics of a test that may guide your studying. The purpose of a test tells you what information the test will cover. The purpose can usually be stated in one to two sentences or phrases. For example, the purpose of a science test may be to assess students' knowledge of the five animal kingdoms. The purpose of a mathematics test may be to determine how well students can solve algebraic equations. No matter how simple or complex, the purpose of a test should be clearly stated and defined (AERA, APA, & NCME, 2004) so that the content on the test is not a mystery to you or any other student. Similarly, the format of a test should be known up front, and should be appropriate for the material being tested (Brennan, 2006). For example, multiple-choice questions work well for a history test that is intended to test historical facts. Essay questions, however, may be more appropriate for a test in a writing class that assesses writing style and grammar. The purpose of this section is help you learn how to study for a test by answering the following question:

- What should I know about the purpose and format of a test?

What should I know about the purpose and format of a test?

Every test has a purpose and format. The purpose or goal of a test should not be a secret kept by your instructor (Broekkamp & van Hout-Wolters, 2007). If the purpose of a test is not clear, you should ask. Similarly, if your instructor has not told you the format of the test, you should ask. There are two main types of question formats: recall and recognition. A recall question asks you to recall information by answering fill-in-the-blank statements or by providing a definition for a term. A recognition question asks you to identify the correct answer to a question. These types of questions may be multiple-choice or true/false. Research has shown that recognition questions tend to be more difficult for students than recall questions (Thiede, 1996). Research has also shown that the expected format of a test affects a student's score more than the anticipated difficulty of a test (Thiede, 1996). In other words, the types of questions you expect to see on a test have a greater impact on your test score than how difficult you anticipate the test being. Whether your instructor uses recall, recognition, or a combination of both types of questions on tests, it is important to learn strategies for answering both types of test questions so that you may improve your test score (Regan, 1977).

 Hands-on strategies

Here are some strategies for studying for a test of any format:

- **Know the purpose of the test.** This will help guide your studying. For example, if the test is about historical facts leading up to World War I, then most (if not all) of your studying should be related to this topic. You shouldn't spend time studying historical facts related to the consequences of the war.

- **Ask the instructor for the format of the exam.** Is it multiple-choice? Essay? Fill-in-the blank? A combination of different formats? This is a fair question and does not give any information away about the content of the test. Knowing the answer to this question will help guide your studying.

- **Practice identifying the parts of test questions.** When you read a test question, you want to be able to identify the introductory information, identify what is being asked, and then identify the information required to answer the question. Practice identifying these parts on questions from your textbook or other resources.

- **Be familiar with test-taking strategies for the format of your test.** There are numerous strategies for answering objective (i.e., multiple-choice) and subjective (i.e., essay) questions. Strategies for two common test formats, multiple-choice and essay are given in Chapter 6 of this book.

Applications

1. Suppose you are enrolled in an English class and just finished reading an assigned novel. The instructor has presented several lectures on the novel and will be giving an exam on the content next week. What do you believe the purpose of the test will be? What will the format of the exam be?

Possible response: One way to answer this question is to write the intended purpose of the test and to think about the exam format most appropriate for that purpose. For example, "The purpose of the test is to assess students' understanding of the facts and lessons presented in the novel." The most appropriate format for this purpose may include multiple-choice items for factual information, and two to three essay questions for comprehension and application questions. Although it is a good exercise to write down the purpose and format that you think is most appropriate, be sure to ask your instructor for the purpose and format, too.

2. Read the multiple-choice question given below and answer parts a through g.

The boy was <u>embbarased</u> after falling off his bicycle.

Which of the following is the correct spelling of the underlined word in the sentence above?
   A. embarrased
   B. embarrassed
   C. embarased
   D. embarassed

Identify the following parts of this multiple-choice question:
   a) purpose of question
   b) stem
   c) question
   d) key words in stem
   e) unimportant information
   f) options
   g) key

Answers to parts a though g:

a) The purpose is to find out if you know how to correctly spell "embbarased"

b) The stem is everything but the options, i.e., "The boy was <u>embbarased</u> after falling off his bicycle. Which of the following is the correct spelling of the underlined word in the sentence above?"

c) "Which of the following is the correct spelling of the underlined word in the sentence above?"

d) embbarased; correct spelling

e) It's not important to know that the boy fell off his bicycle.

f) The options are the four choices you have to choose from.

g) The key is the correct answer. The key in this question is D.

Summary

Every test has a purpose. You should know that purpose. Similarly, there are many different formats for tests and you should know what format to expect on a test. Knowing this information will help you improve your test performance.

 Review

Determine whether statements 1 to 3 are true or false. Select the correct response. Choose the best response to question 4. Answers are provided at the end of this book.

1. True   False   True/False questions are examples of recall questions.

2. True   False   Recognition questions tend to be more difficult than recall questions.

3. True   False   The question format you expect on a test will affect your test score more than the difficulty you expect of the test.

4. Read the multiple-choice question below, then answer the questions.

What is the solution to 5,432 - 2,345?
A. 3,087
B. 3,093
C. 3,113
D. 3,197

    A. What is the purpose of this question?
    B. What is the question?
    C. What is the key?

5.2 Preparing for a test

When should you start studying for a test? Should you study the same way for all tests or should you have different study strategies for different tests? What should you do the day of the test? Evidence suggests that you should begin studying for a test well ahead of time so that you have time to continuously review the material and store the information in your long-term vs. short-term memory (Kornell, 2009; Kitsantas, 2002; Terry 2006). Planning to review your notes, write mock exams, or develop concept maps are just a few strategic examples of ways to plan effective study time (Tinnesz, Ahun, and Kiener, 2006). Including these and other test preparation strategies have proven to increase test performance (Kitsantas, 2002). The purpose of this section is to provide you with strategies that may help you successfully prepare for a test. This section will answer the following question:

- When and how should I study for tests?

When and how should I study for tests?

When should you start studying for a test? Not the night before. "Cramming" for a test has repeatedly shown to be an ineffective way to study for a test (Kornell, 2009; Kistantas, 2002; Rohrer, Taylor, Pashler, Wixted, & Cepeda, 2005). One of the main reasons this is a poor method for studying is because cramming pushes information into your short-term memory that is unavailable in the long term (Terry, 2006). Although your short-term memory may help you with one test or quiz, it is not a good way to help you prepare for comprehensive exams or final exam week, when you have to study and complete multiple comprehensive exams. Research suggests that if you have a plan with study goals, study repeatedly over time, and keep track of (or self-regulate) your learning, your performance in classes will improve (Kistantas, 2002). Studying with peers and constantly asking yourself questions about the materials, such as "How could I explain this to someone?" or "How does this apply to my life or other information I've learned?" may also help you learn the material (van Blerkom, van Blerkom, & Bertsch, 2006; Roberts, 2008; Weinstein, Ridley, Dahl, & Weber, 1988). In addition, as mentioned in Chapter 3, your test scores may increase if you study when you are most alert and your energy and productivity are at their highest levels (Fry, 2005; Lamonte, 2007; Leber, Turk-Browne, & Chun, 2008; Terry, 2006).

 ## Hands-on strategies

Here are a few hands-on strategies that may help you prepare for any test.

- **Schedule your study time.** Write down a schedule for studying and adhere to it. Schedule study time at least two weeks before an exam and at times that you are normally well-rested.

- **Know when tests will occur.** Knowing when to expect tests during the semester or school year will help you plan your studying.

- **Prepare over time, not just the night before.** Don't procrastinate. It is better to have several short study sessions than one or two longer sessions. In addition, early and consistent preparation will reduce test anxiety.

- **Know what information is being tested.** Make sure you know what information to study so you know how to prioritize your studying and do not overlook any topics.

- **Know what to study.** Determine which information is most important and select those parts as the primary targets for your studying and learning.

- **Establish study goals and stick to them.** Once you know what is being tested and what to study, set goals for studying and stick to those goals. Your goals for a test must be thought out and written before you begin your academic endeavors. If you have scheduled 90 minutes of studying for a particular test every other day for two weeks, then stick to that schedule. Don't fall into the trap of procrastinating by telling yourself, "Oh, I'll do it later."

- **Plan time to study alone as well as with other students.** Individual study time is necessary, but teamwork increases brainpower, too. When you explain concepts to others, you will understand the concept better yourself. Others may be able to explain a concept that is unclear to you in a way that makes perfect sense. Group study is good for morale.

- **Plan to review your notes and reread sections of the book you found unclear.** Setting aside time to review your notes and reread sections of the book helps ensure that these important steps are taken. Once you've planned for this review time, follow though with the plan. Chapter 3 offers strategies for everyday learning that can also be applied to studying for a test.

- **If you don't understand, ask.** If there's something you don't understand as you prepare for a test, keep a list and ask someone for help.

- **Plan to answer a set of practice questions about the content.** Practice questions assess and reinforce what you have learned and give you a chance to apply it.

- **Build a positive attitude.** The better your attitude toward studying and learning, the better you'll perform on the test. A positive attitude about studying is a key factor in actually remembering the information.

- **Be an active preparer.** As you review materials, write or type new notes that organize and consolidate information from multiple sources. Not only will this reduce the amount of books, notebooks, and files you'll have to go through for your next review session, but it'll help you learn the information better, too.

- **Arrange your study space.** Collect your class notes, textbooks, and old exams. Organize your pencils, note pads, and highlighter pens. By organizing your study space, you will not have to interrupt your studying to find a necessary study item.

- **Know the type of learner you are and study in ways that complement your learning style.** Chapter 3 offers learning strategies for different learning styles. Once you know your preferred learning style, make sure you use the strategies suggested in that chapter while studying for a test.

Applications

1. The following worksheet may help you prepare for future tests. Adapt the sheet to meet your individual needs.

Preparing for the test
The test is on the following date: _____

I am being tested on: _____

The most important areas for me to study are:
_____
_____

My top 3 goals for studying are:
1. _____
2. _____
3. _____

Resources I will use for studying are:
1. _____
2. _____
3. _____
4. _____

Concepts or examples I don't understand and need to ask someone about are:
1. _____
2. _____
3. _____
4. _____

I can find or create practice questions at the following places or with the following people:
1. _____
2. _____
3. _____

Days and times I have set aside exclusively for studying for this test:
Mondays: _____
Tuesdays: _____
Wednesdays: _____
Thursdays: _____
Fridays: _____
Saturdays: _____
Sundays: _____

2. You are studying for a test with a friend. Your friend is complaining about the class and about studying. Your friend also has notes and books scattered about the table and is clearly flustered by all the material in front of him. As much as you want to have a productive study session, this just isn't happening. What could you say to your friend to make the studying productive?

Possible response: Suggest that your friend stop focusing on the negative parts of studying and the class, and focus on learning the information. In addition, try to find a goal to work toward during your study session. By achieving that goal, your friend may start to have a more positive attitude toward the studying. You may also suggest that your friend organize his notes and books so that only the topics you are reviewing at that particular study session are open. This will help make the studying more focused and the material less overwhelming.

Summary

This section has provided you with several strategies to use when developing a plan for preparing for a test. Some of the most important strategies include studying over a period of time and setting goals for your studying. Once you have a plan in place, the next section will offer strategies for implementing and staying with the plan.

 Review

Determine whether the following statements are true or false. Select the correct response. Answers are provided at the end of this book.

1. True   False   Cramming is a poor method for preparing for a test because the information is stored in your short-term memory only.

2. True   False   Studying alone and with peers is an effective test preparation strategy.

3. True   False   It is important to spend time writing goals for studying.

4. True   False   Creating a mock test with peers is a poor use of time during study sessions.

5.3 Other factors leading to success on a test

Once you have a plan in place for studying for an exam, you need to execute the plan. Executing the plan not only means that you follow through with your study plan, but it also means to treat your body properly so that it is ready to execute your plan. Preparing your body means keeping it healthy with proper food and exercise (Jensen & Nickelsen, 2008). Research has shown that if you maintain good study habits by following through with your plans and also maintaining a healthy lifestyle the days leading up to and the day of the test, then your chances of performing well will be greatest (Cappella, 1982; Chmelynski, 2007). This section will help you execute your plan by answering the following question:

- What do I need to do before the day of the test to ensure success?

What do I need to do before the day of the test to ensure success?

There are several suggestions to keep in mind when executing your study plan. First, remember to study in intervals and not to cram the night before (Kornell, 2009). Cramming will not allow you to get a good night's rest, which is essential before taking an exam. Moreover, if you follow your plan, cramming should not be necessary. Remember to study in intervals, pay attention to what you're learning while studying, review your notes, take mock exams that you make up by yourself or with peers, and review exams that are readily available (Kornell, 2009; Ahuna and Tinnesz, 2003; Tinnesz, Ahuna, & Kiener, 2006).

Your actions the night before the test and the day of the test are crucial to success. Eating breakfast and having a light snack before an exam has proven to increase test performance (Chmelysnki, 2007). The types of snack you want to consume are those that give your brain energy. You want to avoid getting sugar highs or sugar lows — especially during a test. Good brain snacks include low-sugar yogurt, string cheese, graham crackers, fruit, vegetables, pretzels, nuts, or other foods that are low in sugar (Jensen & Nickelsen, 2008). This routine will help your brain and body be in the best shape for performing well on the test.

 Hands-on strategies

The following strategies suggest what to do the night before a test and the day of a test.

- **Assemble everything you will need for the exam the night before.** This may include pencils, erasers, calculators, ID, watch, etc.

- **Get a good night's sleep.** It will help your body function properly during the test.

- **Arrive to the test early.** This will let you find a comfortable place to sit and to not feel rushed immediately before beginning the test.

- **Relax.** You've prepared for the test; now just relax.

- **Use positive affirmations.** You've prepared for the test. Convince yourself by saying, "I have studied well for this test," or "I will do well on this exam."

- **Avoid reviewing content with peers right before the test.** This may cause you to doubt what you have learned.

- **Eat a nutritious snack.** Eat something light and nourishing, not a snack full of sugar.

Application

The following list may help you execute your study plan. Adapt the list as necessary to meet your individual needs.

- When studying
  - Create a study plan similar to that presented in the application portion of Section 5.2
  - Stick to your plan of study
  - Answer the practice questions you found
  - Review your notes and reread sections of the text you found unclear
  - Study alone
  - Study with fellow students
- The night before the test
  - Gather everything you need for the exam (pencils, erasers, ID, calculator, etc.)
  - Get a good night's sleep (don't stay up late studying)
- The day of the test
  - Eat a good breakfast
  - Dress in layers
  - Plan to arrive at the test site early
  - Use the bathroom just before the test
  - Relax
  - Tell yourself that you're ready for the test
  - Do not review content immediately before the test with peers
  - Eat a nourishing snack before taking the test

 Summary

It is one thing to make a study plan; it is another thing to execute it. The execution is the most important part of any plan. Not only do you need to follow your plan, but you need to give your body proper rest and nutrition in the days leading up to and the day of the exam. If you follow the strategies suggested in this chapter, your performance on a test will surely improve. Now that you know how to prepare for a test, the next chapter offers ways to help you increase your score further by providing information and strategies for taking the test.

 Review

Determine whether the following statements are true or false. Select the correct response. Answers are provided at the end of this book.

1. True   False   Peanut butter is a nutritious snack that could be consumed shortly before taking a test to give your brain energy.

2. True   False   It is a good idea to review test material with peers immediately before taking the test.

References

Ahuna, A. H., & Tinnesz, C. G. (2003). *Methods of inquiry: Applied critical thinking.* Dubuque, IA: Kendall/Hunt Publishing.

American Educational Research Association, American Psychological Association, & National Council on Measurement in Education. (2004). *Standards for educational and psychological testing.* Washington DC: American Educational Research Association.

Brennan, R. L. (Ed.). (2006). *Educational measurement* (4th ed.). Westport, CT: Praeger Publishers.

Broekkamp, H., & van Hout-Wolters, B. (2007). Students' adaptation of study strategies when preparing for classroom tests. *Educational Psychology Review, 19*(4), 401-428.

Cappella, B.J., Wagner, M., & Kusmierz, J.A. (1982). Relation of study habits and attitudes to academic performance. *Psychological Reports, 50,* 593–594.

Chmelynski, C. (2007). Free student breakfasts: Surest way to raise performance. *Education Digest, 72*(8), 59-61.

Fry, R. (2005). *How to study.* (6th ed.). Clifton Park, NY: Delmar Learning.

Jensen, E. & Nickelsen, L. (2008). *Deeper learning: 7 powerful strategies for in-depth and longer-lasting learning.* Thousand Oaks, CA: Corwin Press.

Kitsanas, A. (2002). Test preparation and performance: A self-regulatory analysis. *Journal of Experimental Education, 70*(2), 101-13.

Kornell, N. (2009). Optimizing learning using flashcards: Spacing is more effective than cramming. *Applied Cognitive Psychology (in press),* pp. 21.

Lamonte, M. K. (2007). Test-taking strategies for CNOR certification. *Association of Perioperative Registered Nurses, 85*(2), 315-332.

Leber, A. B., Turk-Browne, N. B., & Chun, M. M. (2008). Neural predictors of moment-to-moment fluctuation in cognitive flexibility. *Proceedings of the National Academy of Sciences of the United States of America, 105*(36), 13592-13597.

Regan, J. (1977). Strategies in learning for recall and recognition tests. *The American Journal of Psychology, 90*(2), 313—318.

Rohrer, D., Taylor, K., Pashler, H., Wixted, J. T., & Cepeda, N. J. (2005). The effect of overlearning on long-term retention. *Applied Cognitive Psychology, 19,* 361-374.

Roberts, D. (2008). Learning in clinical practice: The importance of peers. *Nursing Standard, 23*(12), 35-41.

Terry, W. S. (2006). *Learning and memory* (3rd ed.). Boston: Pearson Education, Inc.

Thiede, K. W. (1996). The relative importance of anticipated test format and anticipated test difficulty on performance. *The Quarterly Journal of Experimental Psychology, 49A*(4), 901-918.

Tinnesz, C., Ahuna, K., & Kiener, M. (2006). Toward college success: Internalizing active and dynamic strategies. *College Teaching, 54*(4), 302-306.

Van Blerkhom, D. L., van Blerkhom, M. L., & Bertsch S. (2006). Study strategies and generative learning: What works? *Journal of College Reading and Learning, 37*(1), 7-18.

Weinstein, C. E., Ridley, D. S., Dahl, T., & Weber, E. S. (1988). Helping students develop strategies for effective learning. *Educational Leadership, 46*(4), 17-19.

Although the goal of any assessment is to find out whether or not you have mastered the presented material, tests sometimes inadvertently test nonacademic areas. For example, a test will not be an accurate representation of how much you know about a subject if your performance is hurt by test anxiety. If you are so nervous about the test that you forget information during the test that you know you have learned, then the test is being negatively affected by the nonacademic feeling of anxiety. On the other hand, sometimes nerves or other nonacademic factors can be countered by knowing some general test-taking strategies, as well as some specific strategies for taking multiple-choice and essay tests. By applying these strategies, you may be able to jog your memory and recall the information that your anxiety blocked. Even if you have no test anxiety, knowing some of the strategies presented in this chapter can improve your test performance.

6.1 Dealing with test anxiety

Test anxiety can affect people at different times and in different ways. Some people become anxious about tests several weeks before actually taking them, others have trouble sleeping the night before, and still others draw a blank during the test. These and many other examples describe ways anxiety can affect test performance. The purpose of this section is to provide answers to the following questions:

- What is test anxiety? Who is affected by it? Are there ways to reduce it?

What is test anxiety? Who is affected by it? Are there ways to reduce it?

Do you experience difficulty sleeping the night before a test? Do you have difficulty concentrating while taking a test? Do you worry about running out of time to finish a test? Do you draw a blank to the answer to a test question that you know you can answer? When you are taking a test, do you find your heart beating faster? If you answered "yes" to any of these questions, then you may be experiencing test anxiety. Although it is normal to feel a little nervous and stressed before a test, researchers have projected that nearly 10 million pre-college students struggle with test anxiety (Hill & Wigfield, 1984; McDonald, 2001).

What is test anxiety? Test anxiety is a fear of performing poorly on tests (Beidel, Turner & Taylor-Ferreira, 1999). The higher your anxiety level, the worse you will perform (Hancock, 2001). Test anxiety can impair your ability to solve problems and answer more difficult questions because it limits your brain's ability to recall learned material (Eysenck, 1979, 1981; Hasher & Zucks, 1988; Tobias, 1985).

 Hands-on strategies

If you are experiencing test anxiety during the test, the following strategies may help:

- **Breathe.** If you begin to feel nervous, slowly take a few deep breaths and return to work.

- **Relax.** The more relaxed you are, the less likely you'll have memory lapses during the test.

- **Visualize.** Think about a peaceful place, tell yourself that you came prepared for this test, or imagine receiving this test back with a good grade.

- **Be positive.** Give yourself words of encouragement, such as "I'm well-prepared for the test" or "I can do this!"

- **Immediately write down memorized information.** When you receive the test, immediately write down formulas, definitions, and key words in the margins so that you don't have to worry about forgetting these facts.

- **Answer simple questions first.** Answering the easier questions first will help build your confidence and help you tackle more difficult questions later on.

- **Don't get discouraged.** Remember that you don't have to get every question right to do well.

 Applications

1. You and a friend have studied for a biology test together. When you go to the test, you are both confident that you are prepared and knowledgeable about the content that the test will cover. During the test, you notice that your friend is sweating and restless. You hear her mumble under her breath, "I know the answer. Why can't I come up with it now?" After the test, she is clearly frustrated and tells you that she did not do well on the test. Give 3 to 5 suggestions that you could offer to your friend to help her control her test anxiety for the next test.

Possible response: Your response to your friend may include, among other suggestions, that she take some deep breaths during the test to help her relax. You may also suggest that she visualize doing well on the test since she was prepared for the test and knew the content. Also, encourage her to remain positive throughout the testing process. Remind her she is able to earn a good grade, but that she has to believe in herself first.

2. After taking several tests in a history class, you realize that you are losing points over factual questions. These "easy points" that you are losing cause you to lose focus on the more difficult questions which have more points associated with them. What could you do to improve your performance on the next test?

Possible response: Because the problem is associated with memorized facts, try writing down as many memorized facts in the margins of your test as soon as it is given to you. Although it may take some time to write down these facts, they will probably save you time in the long run because you won't have to try to recall the facts if and when they appear on the test. Moreover, this will help ensure that you get the "easy points" and allow your brain to focus on the more difficult questions. Also, remember that it is usually possible to miss a couple of questions and still do well on a test.

3. If you experience test anxiety, try the following steps the next time you enter a classroom to take a test:

- **Step 1.** Try to arrive at the testing location as early as possible.

- **Step 2.** Promptly find your seat and prepare your test-taking materials.

- **Step 3.** Relax your mind before the test by following the breathing procedure below. You can use this procedure during the test or whenever you feel anxious. The technique only takes a few seconds and it can make your test session less stressful.

  - First, sit up straight.

  - Second, close your eyes. Slowly inhale by closing your mouth and inhaling through your nose. Visualize filling your lower lungs with air, then your upper lungs.

  - Next, hold your breath for a few seconds, and then exhale slowly through your mouth.

  - Finally, wait a few seconds, and then repeat this process.

- **Step 4.** Relax your body before the test by following the technique described below.

  - First, place your arms at your side.

  - Next, close your eyes.

  - Tense your forehead muscles for about 10 seconds, then let them completely relax. Continue to tense and relax muscles starting with your head and working your way down to your toes. As you do this, concentrate on making the muscles relax more and more.

  - Finally, wait 20 seconds, and then repeat this process.

 Summary

Test anxiety is relatively common. Research has shown it can impair test performance by limiting your ability to concentrate and recall memory. However, you can minimize test anxiety by learning to relax both before and during a test.

 Review

Determine if the following statements are true or false. Select the correct response. Answers are provided at the end of this book.

1. True   False   Test anxiety is rare among students.

2. True   False   Anxiety can influence our ability to recall memory.

3. True   False   Anxiety can influence our ability to concentrate.

4. True   False   It is possible to identify the symptoms of test anxiety.

6.2 General test-taking strategies

The purpose of this section is to introduce and familiarize you with general test-taking strategies. More strategies are suggested in sections 6.3 and 6.4 for multiple-choice and essay tests, respectively. For this section, the focus is on time management and reading directions. Specifically, this section can help you become a more knowledgeable and savvy test-taker by answering the following questions:

- What are some time management strategies that I can follow while taking a test?

- Should I read the directions and know how the questions are scored?

What are some time management strategies that I can follow while taking a test?

Good time management skills are essential. Not surprisingly, they can be a very important part of the test-taking process. Research has shown that students who perform well on tests typically take the time to assess the length and difficulty of a test before starting (Hong, Sas, & Sas, 2006), while those who lack time management skills perform worse (Gulek, 2003).

 Hands-on strategies

If you feel that your time management skills could be improved during tests, you may consider adopting some of the strategies listed here.

- **Use a watch.** Pace yourself and set goals for completing the test. About halfway through the test, check your watch to ensure that you are on track for finishing on time.

- **Review the test before starting.** Try to determine how much time you will spend on each section (e.g., multiple-choice, matching, and essay). Remember, essay questions usually require more time.

- **I'm stuck, what next?** Try not to stay on one question too long, especially if the question is not worth many points. Skip ahead to questions you know that you can readily answer, and then go back to the more difficult ones later.

- **Extra time?** Don't try to impress anyone by finishing first. Your grade is based on your answers, not on how quickly you finish the test. If you have extra time, check your answers.

Should I read the directions and know how the questions are scored?

Are you someone who skips to the first question on a test without reading the directions? Not surprisingly, this type of mistake can affect your test performance dramatically. It is strongly recommended that you read and clearly understand what you are being asked to do on a test, as well as understand how the test will be scored (Ellis & Ryan, 2003). A good set of directions will provide information about how you should record your answers and the scoring procedures that will be used (Thorndike, 1997).

 Hands-on strategies

The following are some hands-on strategies to help you navigate through the directions and scoring procedures on a test.

- **Assess point values.** Identify the point values associated with each question. Budget the appropriate amount of time to answer questions with the greatest point values.

- **Look for special information.** Are you supposed to answer all of the questions, or only a portion?

- **Clarify uncertainties.** Ask the instructor if you don't understand the directions, a question, or the scoring.

- **Stay focused.** Answer the question being asked. Respond to questions based on the information provided in the question.

- **Look for key words.** Underline phrases in the stem or responses that make questions negative (e.g., not, except, false). Look for specific determiners or words that mean something absolute or definite (e.g., always, never).

- **Order matters.** If a question addresses the order of an event, pay attention to words that indicate sequence (e.g., first, before, later, next).

 Applications

1. A student took a test with a time limit of one hour. The test consisted of two short essays worth 15 points each, one long essay question worth 40 points, and 30 multiple-choice items worth one point each. The student finished the first two essay questions, but failed to finish the third essay and the multiple choice questions within the provided time limit. The student spent the following amount of time on each question:

   Essay 1 (15 points) – 30 minutes
   Essay 2 (15 points) – 15 minutes
   Essay 3 (40 points) – 5 minutes
   30 multiple choice questions (30 points) – 10 minutes

What did this student do wrong? What would you recommend this student do next time?

Possible Response: The student should review the point values and the number of items on the test before beginning. If time were managed correctly, the student should have spent about 40% of the time on Essay 3 (or about 24 minutes), 30% of the time on the multiple choice questions (or about 18 minutes), and the remaining time split evenly between Essay 1 and Essay 2. By not managing time appropriately, this student missed several multiple-choice questions that could have been answered quickly and correctly.

2. Read each of the following sets of directions. For each set, underline the key words. What important information might you miss if you did not read the directions carefully? Is there additional information you might want to know before answering the questions?

   A. Ten statements are given below. Decide whether each statement is true or false and circle your response. If the statement is false, cross out the incorrect part of the statement and write in the necessary information to make the statement true. You only need to complete 8 of these questions. Each question is worth 2 points.

   B. Describe in 500 words or less how to test the acidity level of a solution. (5 points)

   C. In 5 to 6 paragraphs, summarize Stephen King's novel *The Shining*. Be sure to describe the main characters, setting, and plot (6 points).

   D. List four reasons why you should not study for a test the night before taking it.

Possible responses: A. If you did not read these directions carefully, you might miss that you only need to complete 8 of the 10 questions and that you need to correct the false statements.

B. If you did not read these directions carefully, you might miss that you have a 500-word limit and that you are supposed to describe "how," i.e. what steps are needed, to test the acidity level.

C. If you did not read these directions carefully, you might miss that there are three items that must be discussed and that you have a 5 to 6 paragraph limit.

D. If you did not read these directions carefully, you might miss the word "not." You may also need to ask the instructor for clarification as to whether the question is supposed to be "only the night before" or "the night before" in general, which may not make much sense. You might also want to know the point value associated with this question.

Summary

Test-taking strategies can be very useful and easy to implement. If used correctly, they can help you relax, improve your time management skills, and ultimately become a smarter test-taker. You will probably perform better on your next test if you take the time to learn about the test before starting. In addition, you should clearly understand what you are being asked to do on a test as well as to review the scoring procedures.

 Review

Answer question 1. For questions 2 and 3, determine if the statements are true or false. Select the correct response. Answers are provided at the end of this book.

1. List four time management skills that you could use while taking a test.

2. True   False   Students can learn how to become better test-takers.

3. True   False   Most students read the directions and scoring procedures on a test.

6.3 Test-taking strategies for multiple-choice tests

Have you ever wondered why multiple choice questions are so difficult? After all, the answer is there in front of you — right? Yes, but tempting wrong answers are staring back at you as well. Although you may know the answer to a question, the wrong answers may make you second-guess yourself. The purpose of this section is to help you ferret though the distractors and focus on the correct response by answering the following question:

- How do I eliminate response options on a multiple-choice test?

How do I eliminate response options on a multiple-choice test?

The most common selected-response format used in college classrooms is multiple-choice (Jacobs & Chase, 1992). Learning specific test-taking strategies for taking multiple-choice tests may improve your overall test performance by providing strategies that may help you eliminate response choices (Paris et al., 1991). For example, if a question has four potential options (i.e., A, B, C, or D), you automatically have a 25% chance of selecting the correct answer. However, if you can eliminate one or more of the four response options, you have a better chance of selecting the correct answer.

 Hands-on strategies

The following strategies may help you learn to eliminate response options or decide which options to select.

- **Rule out wrong answers.** By using your existing knowledge, you may be able to identify an incorrect answer. If so, place an "X" through the answer and focus on the remaining choices.

- **Cover up the choices and answer the question.** The choices may make you second-guess yourself. If you know the answer without looking at the choices, then choose the option closest to your answer and don't second-guess yourself by reading the distractors.

- **Recognize opposite response options.** On a classroom test, if you find two opposite response choices, one is probably correct.

- **Watch for "all of the above."** If you can clearly eliminate a response choice, then you have already determined that an "all of the above" response choice is not the correct answer. Conversely, if you can identify that two responses are correct, and "all of the above" is an option, choose it.

- **Look for absolute words.** On a classroom test, look for words that tend to make statements incorrect (e.g., always, never, all, only, must, and will). Statements using absolute or definite words tend to be incorrect because they do not apply in all situations.

- **Make educated guesses.** If you can't decide which response choice is best, make an educated guess.

- **Work backwards.** Sometimes, you may have more success in answering a question by looking at the options first and working backwards. This technique is especially useful in math questions.

 Applications

Answer each multiple-choice question based on your general knowledge and the strategies listed in this section.

1. The United States' Civil War began in which of the following years?

    A. 1776
    B. 1781
    C. 1861
    D. 1865

The correct answer is C. If you didn't know that the Civil War began in 1861, your knowledge may at least help you rule out options A and B. By eliminating these two options, you now have a 50-50 chance of selecting the correct answer. On the other hand, maybe you knew the answer was 1861, but the option of 1865 made you second-guess yourself. Trust your instincts.

2. Which of the following statements about shapes is true?

        A. A square is a rectangle.

        B. A rectangle is a square.

        C. A trapezoid is a rhombus.

        D. A trapezoid is a rectangle.

The correct answer is A. If you didn't know the answer to this problem, you could look at the options and see that A and B are opposites. As long as C and D are not opposites, too, it would be reasonable to guess that the answer is either A or B.

3. Which of the following are primary colors?

        A. Red

        B. Yellow

        C. Blue

        D. All of the above

The correct answer is D. If you knew at least two of the primary colors, you would immediately know that the correct answer is D.

4. Which of the following facts is true about bats?

        A. All bats have fur.

        B. Bats are a type of bird.

        C. Most bats live in tropical forests.

        D. Nutrient needs remain the same throughout a bat's life.

The correct answer is C. Option A uses the absolute word "all." Option D uses the phrase "remain the same," which is equivalent to saying "never change." "Never" is another absolute word. It is rare that the correct answer to a multiple-choice question will be one that uses an absolute word, because it is unlikely for something to always occur or to never occur. Options A and B are both plausible, but B is incorrect because bats are mammals.

5. Lucy Maud Montgomery's novel, *Anne of Green Gables,* is written primarily from which of the following characters' points of view?

        A. Anne

        B. Marilla

        C. Matthew

        D. Diana

The correct answer is A. Even if you have not read this novel, the title may lead you to make an educated guess that the main character is Anne and that the story is most likely told from her perspective.

6. Which of the following integers is a solution to the equation $2x^2 - 3 = x$?

        A. -2

        B. -1

        C. 1

        D. 2

The correct answer is B. If you didn't know how to solve this problem, you could insert each integer into the equation and see which one works. The only integer that solves this equation is -1.

Summary

Multiple-choice questions are commonly used in college classrooms. Take the time to learn the common rules and procedures used to solve multiple-choice test questions because it may improve your score on a test. These rules may help you eliminate response choices and improve your chances of correctly answering a question.

 Review

Select the correct response to each of the following questions. Answers are provided at the end of this book.

1. Which of the following types of selected-response questions are most commonly used in college classrooms?

    A. Fill-in-the-blank
    B. True/False
    C. Matching
    D. Multiple-choice

2. Which of the following words tends to make statements incorrect in a multiple-choice question?

    A. All
    B. Some
    C. A few
    D. Many

3. After a reading a four-option multiple choice question, you are able to eliminate one option. What are your chances of guessing the correct response after this elimination?

    A. 25%
    B. 33%
    C. 50%
    D. 66%

6.4 Test-taking strategies for essay tests

Do you have a set of strategies for writing an essay test? If so, are they effective? Do you know what your instructor or some other grader is looking for when he or she grades your test? The purpose of this section is to provide test-taking strategies for responding to essay questions on tests. Keep in mind as you read this section that there are two types of essay questions: long and short. A long essay question may ask: "Trace the history of events that led up to World War I" or "Compare and contrast Shakespeare's *Romeo and Juliet* with *Hamlet*. How are they similar? How are they different?" A short essay question could ask: "In a well-organized paragraph, explain Poe's theory of poetry" or "List the major provisions of a treaty and briefly explain the significance of each one." Whichever type of essay question you have, the hands-on strategies provided in this section should help you become a better essay test-taker. The purpose of this section is to answer the following question:

- What are some strategies for taking essay tests?

What are some strategies for taking essay tests?

Instructors use essay questions because they are useful for measuring how well you can organize, integrate, and express ideas (Gronlund, 2003). When composing an essay by hand, use legible handwriting and avoid spelling or grammatical errors. Research has demonstrated that a legible essay response will be assigned a significantly higher grade than will a non-legible essay response (Marshall & Powers, 1969). Further, essay responses containing spelling or grammatical errors are assigned significantly lower grades than are essay responses containing no major composition errors (Marshall & Powers, 1969).

 Hands-on strategies

The following strategies offer tips that may help you improve your score on your next essay test.

- **Be familiar with commonly used words in essay questions.** If you know what key words are often asked in an essay question, then you won't have to spend time thinking about their meaning during the test (see Application 1 of this section).

- **Complete pre-writing activities.** To help you focus and prepare to write an essay, be sure to take the time to do the following:

    o **Review the test to determine how much time you can spend on each question.** See which questions you should answer first or last, which ones are worth the most points, and how much time you should allot to each question.

    o **Manage your time.** Plan how much time you will spend on each question and write it down after reviewing the test. Wear a watch and keep track of how much time you have spent on each essay question and how much time you have remaining.

    o **Read the directions to make sure you understand what is being asked.** If it helps, restate the question in your own words. When reading the directions, underline key words or questions. Besides content, read the directions to determine whether you can select the essays you want to answer or if you have to answer all of the questions. Also, see if the directions specify point values or required lengths. If you have questions, be sure to ask the instructor for clarification.

    o **Make a brief outline to organize and clarify your thoughts.** List key words and concepts in or beside your outline. This will keep them available later when pressure and anxiety may otherwise block them. If you don't have time to finish, you can refer to your outline and potentially earn partial credit. Teachers appreciate a compact, clear, and well-organized answer.

- **Be as clear as possible when writing.** The reader of your essay will be impressed if you answer the question directly, with clarity, and without unnecessary information. Do the following:

    o **Use examples to support and explain your points.**

    o **Write succinctly.** Define terms, explain statements, and support ideas with facts. Instructors are usually impressed by brevity and accuracy.

    o **Write with visual aids to guide the reader.** Include headings, numbering, and line spacing in your writing so that it is easy to read.

- **Structure your essays.** Follow your outline and support it with main ideas, facts, illustrations, and examples. Ensure that your essay has the following components:

  o **An introduction which states your main point(s)** — The introduction will often be your "thesis" statement. If you initially can't develop one, leave a few blank lines so you can fill it in later.

  o **Topic sentences highlighting the main idea beginning each paragraph** — The rest of the paragraph should include details that support the topic sentence (i.e., facts, dates and examples).

  o **Transitional words that will improve the flow and clarity of your writing** — Use words such as first, second, moreover, in addition, also, however, finally, and therefore.

  o **A summary and conclusion which ends the essay** — A summary is simply a paraphrase of the introduction and a conclusion states your final thoughts or comments on the essay as a whole.

- **Don't be in a hurry to turn in your work.** After you have finished writing, reread the question and proofread your work for the following:

  o **You answered all questions.** Be certain you answered what was asked. Have you left out any words or parts of answers? Have you attempted every question? If you have no idea of the correct answer, write something related. Partial credit is better than zero credit. If you run out of time, try writing a partial response or outline rather than leaving the question blank. Always write something. If you don't know the answer, try to reason it out.

  o **You said everything you wanted to say.** Have you covered everything in your outline? If you haven't said everything pertinent to answering the question and you still have time, then add it.

  o **Your writing is organized.** Make sure your essay is easy to read and to follow.

  o **Your essay is free of spelling and grammar mistakes and your handwriting is legible.** Multiple spelling or grammar errors are not impressive and hurts the overall presentation of your essay. Similarly, illegible writing hurts the flow of your paper and makes it difficult for the reader to know what you are trying to say.

Applications

1. There are several common verbs used in essay questions. Understanding these verbs and their associated meanings is essential to becoming a better test-taker.

Develop an essay question using the common verbs in Table 6.1. Provide specific directions regarding how to respond to the questions as well as how you will assign point values. Keep in mind that a good set of directions will provide information about how the examinees are to record their answers, the basis on which they are to select their answers, and the scoring procedures that will be used.

COMMON ESSAY VERBS	MEANING
Analyze	Divide into parts, then examine, discuss, or interpret each part separately and as a whole.
Compare/Contrast	Explain the similarities and differences. Comparisons usually ask for similarities more than differences.
Criticize	Analyze an issue or issues and state your opinion about the correctness or value of that issue. Make judgments about quality or worth (positive and negative).
Define	Explain the meaning. Give enough detail to demonstrate understanding. Definitions are usually short. Be sure to give word context so that it is distinguishable from similar words.
Describe	Give a detailed account of an event or quality, including who, what, where, when, and why. Include a list of characteristics.
Diagram	Draw a picture and label the parts. Discuss the relevant and procedural processes.
Discuss	Investigate by reason or argument. Debate the pros and cons of an issue. Consider various points of view.
Enumerate	List or write down in a succinct form several ideas, concepts, events, reasons, or other necessary information.
Evaluate	React logically to a topic. Discuss the strengths and weaknesses of a topic. State your opinion or provide a citation of another person's opinion. Provide evidence that supports the stated opinion.
Explain	Provide facts and details to clarify an idea or concept. Discuss who, what, where, when, and why.
Illustrate	Explain a concept with clear examples, diagrams, charts, or pictures.
Interpret	Translate or describe the meaning of a concept or relationship.
Justify	Provide reasons to support an action, event, or policy. Present evidence or facts to support a position.
List/Name	Make a brief list.
Outline	Explain the main ideas, characteristics, or events.
Prove	Establish a position, concept, or theory by using facts, evidence, and logic.
State	Explain precisely.
Summarize	Cover the major points in a concise manner. Omit unnecessary details.
Trace	Chronologically describe the development or progress of a particular trend, event, or process.

Table 6.1 Common Essay Verbs and Their Meaning

2. One of the best ways to study for an essay test is to write practice essays. As you practice your next essay, use the list below as a guideline for writing a succinct, error-proof essay that answers the question(s) posed.

- Before you start writing

  o Review the questions and estimate the order and amount of time you will dedicate to answering each of the questions.

  o Read all directions.

  o Outline your writing.

- While writing

  o Use examples.

  o Be concise and to the point.

  o Use appropriate vocabulary terms (if applicable).

    ○   Spend the amount of time you allotted to each question — not more.

    ○   Use headings, numbering, and/or use space so your paper is easy to read.

    ○   Structure your essay.

        ■   Introduction

        ■   Topic sentences

        ■   Transitional words

        ■   Summary and conclusion

    ○   Proofread.

        ■   All parts of all questions are answered

        ■   Answers complete

        ■   Writing is organized

        ■   Writing has no known spelling or grammar errors

        ■   All writing is legible

 ## Summary

Before writing, take a few minutes to review and learn about the essay. This will help you decide where to start and how much time to spend on each question. It will be helpful to understand the common verbs used in essay tests and their associated meanings. When composing an essay by hand, remember to use legible handwriting and avoid spelling or grammatical errors. Research has demonstrated that a legible essay response will be assigned a significantly higher grade than will a non-legible essay response. Also, essay responses containing spelling or grammatical errors were assigned significantly lower grades than were essay responses containing no major composition errors. Lastly, use the feedback from the test to improve your test-taking strategies.

 ## Review

Determine if the statements in questions 1 and 2 are true or false. Select the correct response. Follow the instructions in question 3. Select the best option for questions 4 to 7. Answers are provided at the end of this book.

1. True   False   Spelling and grammar are not important when writing an essay.

2. True   False   Questions worth more points should be allotted more time.

3. Name some important parts of an essay that give it overall structure.

4. Which of the following verbs found in an essay question means that you should describe the main events, characteristics, or events?

    A. Diagram
    B. Evaluate
    C. Outline
    D. Prove

5. Which of the following verbs found in an essay question means that you should write about different points of view?

    A. Define
    B. Discuss
    C. Illustrate
    D. Trace

6. Which of the following verbs found in an essay question means that you should separate an idea into several parts and examine each part?

      A. Analyze

      B. Compare

      C. Justify

      D. Summarize

7. Which of the following verbs found in an essay question means that you should explain a concept as accurately and precisely as possible?

      A. Criticize

      B. Describe

      C. Enumerate

      D. State

References

Beidel, D.C., Turner, S. M. & Taylor-Ferreira, J. C. (1999). Teaching study skills and test-taking strategies to elementary school students: The testbusters program. *Behavior Modification, 23* (4), 630-646.

Ellis, A. P. J. & Ryan, A. M. (2003). Race and cognitive-ability test performance: The mediating effects of test preparation, test-taking strategy use and self-efficacy. *Journal of Applied Social Psychology, 33*(12), 2607-2629.

Eysenck, H. J. (1981). *A model for personality.* Berlin: Springer.

Eysenck, M. W. (1979). Anxiety, learning and memory: A reconceptualization. *Journal of Research in Personality, 13,* 363-385.

Gronlund, N. E. (2003). *Assessment of student achievement* (7th ed.). Boston: Allyn & Bacon.

Gulek, C. (2003). Preparing for high-stakes testing. *Theory into Practice, 42*(1), 42-50.

Hancock, D.R. (2001). Effects of test anxiety and evaluative threat on students' achievement and motivation. *The Journal of Educational Research, 94*(5), 284- 290.

Hasher, L. & Zacks, R. T. (1988). Working memory, comprehension, and aging: A review and a new view. *The Psychology of Learning and Motivation, 22,* 193-225.

Hill, K., & Wigfield, A. (1984). Test anxiety: A major educational problem and what can be done about it. *Elementary School Journal, 85,* 105-126.

Hong, E., Sas, M., & Sas, J. C. (2006). Test-taking strategies of high and low mathematics achievers. *Journal of Educational Research, 99*(3), 144-155.

Jacobs, L. C., & Chase, C. I. (1992). *Developing and using tests effectively: A guide for faculty.* San Francisco, CA: Josey-Bass.

Marshall, J. C. & Powers, J. M. (1969). Writing neatness, composition errors and essay grades. *Journal of Educational Measurement, 6*(2), 97-101. National Council on Measurement in Education.

McDonald, A. S. (2001). The prevalence and effects of test anxiety in school children. *Educational Psychology, 21*(1), 89-101.

Paris, S. G., Lawton, T. A., Turner, J. C., & Roth, J. L. (1991). A developmental perspective on standardized achievement testing. *Educational Researcher, 20*(5), 12-20.

Thorndike, R. M. (1997). *Measurement and evaluation in psychology and education.* Prentice Hall: Upper Saddle River, New Jersey

Tobias, S. (1985). Test anxiety: Interference, defective skills and cognitive capacity. *Educational Psychologist, 20*(3), 135-142.

You have studied and taken the test. This chapter offers some suggestions to follow if you did not achieve your desired score. This chapter also discusses ways for you to remember the information you learned.

7.1 Tips to consider if you did not achieve your desired score

Did you achieve the score you wanted on a test? If so, congratulations. The test-taking and study strategies you used worked. If not, you're not alone. If you did not receive the score you hoped to achieve, re-evaluate your study and test-taking strategies. Which strategies worked? Which ones did not? Research suggests that the more active strategies you implement into your studying, the better your performance in that class (Gettinger & Seibert, 2002). This section will provide strategies for improving your study habits if you did not achieve the test score you expected by answering the following question:

- What can I do to improve my score?

What can I do to improve my score?

This book has offered a wide range of strategies for studying and test-taking that is supported by research. If you have not achieved your desired score, review the chapters in this book for alternative study and test-taking strategies. If you feel that these strategies are still not working, consider other factors that may be contributing to your performance. If you are also working while going to school, for example, you may want to reconsider the number of hours or time of day that you work. Research is mixed about whether working helps or hinders academic performance, but some have found that students who work do not do as well in class as students who do not work (Stinebrickner & Stinebrickner, 2003). It is not clear, however, whether this trend holds for students beyond their first semester in college (Ruhm, 1997). If you are not working or if you cannot reduce the number of hours or change the time of day you are working, your school counselor may be able to offer more individualized strategies for you.

 Hands-on strategies

Consider the following hands-on strategies if you think you need to change your study habits or need other suggestions for improving your test score:

- **Implement new study strategies immediately.** If you are unhappy with your results, try a new study strategy and implement it immediately. Evaluate its success after the next test.

- **Join a study group.** If you normally study alone, consider studying with fellow students. If you are already involved in a study group, try studying with a different group of students.

- **Spend individual time studying.** Plan to spend some time studying by yourself. After all, you are not taking the test as a group.

- **If you are in a study group, assess how the group uses the study time.** Is the group mainly on task or are there a lot of side conversations?

- **Seek other sources, including non-text sources.** If the information you are required to know is not clear in your notes or text, seek out another textbook, search the Internet, ask the instructor, or look for audiotapes, videos, DVDs, or CDs available on the topic to enhance your learning.

- **Test your knowledge.** Review test questions in your textbook or other resources, or try writing and answering test questions for people in your study group (if you use one).

- **Ask yourself questions that reinforce your learning.** For example, "If I had to teach this concept to another student, how would I explain it?" or "If someone asked me to summarize this concept, what would I say?"

- **Ask your instructor to explain questions on the test you missed and don't understand.** If you leave a test and still feel like you do not understand an important concept, make an appointment to discuss the concept with the instructor.

- **Consult a school counselor if you are experiencing test anxiety and cannot control it.** If you are feeling a lot of anxiety before and during a test, your school counselor may be able to provide you with some extra tips for overcoming the anxiety.

- **Re-evaluate your work and extracurricular schedule.** If you are working or have extracurricular activities, consider reducing your hours at these activities so that you can spend more time studying. Alternatively, try changing the hours of your activities so that you study when you are most alert.

Applications

1. A first-year college student received her history test back and was disappointed with her performance. She thought she prepared for the exam properly. When studying for the exam, she made diagrams of historical events because she knew she was a visual learner. She watched some extra videos about the historical events that she knew would be on the test. In addition, she created flashcards to help her remember dates and started reviewing these flash cards the night before the exam. Preferring to study alone, she studied at the library every night for two weeks before the exam. The night before the exam, she worked a job from 5 to 10 p.m. When she got home, she studied until 1 a.m. The day of the exam, she awoke at 5:30 a.m. to study some more. She drank two cans of regular cola at 8 a.m., ate a bowl of cereal with a banana at 8:30 a.m., and then went to class to take the exam. She arrived at the classroom at 8:45 a.m. and the test began at 9 a.m. She chatted with her friends before the test, but refused to talk about any of the material related to the test. Despite all her preparation, she ended up with a C on the test. What did this student do correctly? What could she do to improve her score on the next test?

Possible response: What she did correctly:

Made diagrams

Watched videos (an additional resource) to help her learn or reinforce the material

Created flashcards

Studied alone (as noted below, she should also consider group study)

Ate a healthy breakfast prior to the exam (no need for snack since the exam was 30 minutes after she ate breakfast)

Refused to talk about the test material with her peers immediately before the exam

What she could do to improve:

Review the flashcards several times before the exam; not just the night before

Try studying with peers

Avoid working the night before a test

Only study until 8 or 9 p.m. to ensure a good night sleep before the test day

Drink milk or water or a cup of juice instead of regular soda; lots of sugar should be avoided before taking a test

2. Is your study group effective? Try using the following list when studying in a group. If you are able to check all of the boxes, then your study group is off to a good start.

☐ My study group spends less than 10% of the time on side conversations.

☐ In my study group, we spend a lot of time explaining concepts and summarizing concepts to each other.

☐ In my study group, we make sure that everyone understands the errors that were made on the last exam.

☐ If no one in my study group knows the answer to a question, we either look it up or someone asks the instructor.

☐ If we notice one of our study group members is very knowledgeable about the subject, but is performing poorly on the tests, we discuss non-academic reasons for his performance. If it sounds like he is anxious about tests, we might suggest he talk to a counselor to figure out ways to deal with anxiety.

Summary

This section has offered a few tips to help troubleshoot study and test-taking problems not previously addressed in this book. Specifically, this section has suggested that you look at your work or extracurricular schedule or perhaps visit a school counselor to figure out what measures you should take to improve your test scores if you are not happy with your performance.

 Review

Determine whether the first statement below is true or false. Select the correct response. Supply responses for the second question. Answers are provided at the end of this book.

1. True   False   Working while in school lowers academic performance.

2. If you have not achieved your desired test score, what are three strategies that you could try implementing for the next test?

      1. _____

      2. _____

      3. _____

7.2 Retaining the information learned

You have studied for your test, taken the test, and are ready to start the cycle over again with new material. After taking the test, however, you don't want to lose the information you learned for the test. Whether or not you find the information interesting or useful, you will most likely come across the same information on your final exam or in another course. So, how do you retain the information learned? The simple answer is to continue to review the material (Howe & Branierd, 1989). Review the feedback your instructor gave you on previous tests, review your notes periodically, and find ways to integrate the information you learned into the new information being presented (Kang, McDermott, & Roediger, 2007; Terry 2006; Jensen & Nickelsen, 2008). Using these strategies and others, this section will help suggest ways to answer the following question:

- How do I retain the information I learned for a test?

How do I retain the information I learned for a test?

Your instructor has just returned your test. You see your score and then bury the test in a folder with other class papers. Do you ever plan on looking at the test again? If you hope to retain the information you learned from studying for the test, you should. Research has shown that reviewing the feedback an instructor provides on a test directly correlates to improved test performance (Kang, McDermott, Roediger, 2007). Moreover, revisiting the information by either retaking the test or taking self-tests of the information will help you retain the information over a longer period of time (Howe, Branierd, 1989). Not only will this type of reviewing help with long-term memory retention, but it will help you learn new information that builds on the knowledge you just learned. In other words, old information primes your mind for new information just like a movie preview primes your desire to watch the movie (Jensen and Nickelsen, 2008; Terry 2006).

 Hands-on strategies

The following list of suggestions may help you retain the information learned from studying for a test.

- **Reward yourself.** You learned the information for a test, now take a break and reward yourself. The more positive the testing experience, the better you'll be prepared to start studying for the next test.

- **Look up any questions that you couldn't answer.** Once you've had time to relax, go back and look up any information on the test that you didn't know. You're more likely to retain that information when you're in a relaxed state and have time to dedicate to learning it.

- **Review mistakes.** Once you get a test back, be sure to go back and find out what you did wrong on any questions that you missed. Be sure you know what the correct answer is.

- **Read feedback.** If your instructor has taken the time to write feedback on a test, read it. If you don't understand what the instructor has written, then ask for clarification.

- **Continue to review the information.** The phrase, "Use it or lose it" has merit. Continue to review the information you learned for the test. The more you review it, the more likely it will stay in your long-term memory. In addition, every time you review it, you will probably understand it better.

- **Teach concepts to others.** Other students will be tested on the same material or may not have understood it as well as you. Offer to tutor students. By explaining the concept to others, you will retain it longer and learn it better yourself.

Application

Read the following list. Check the statements you believe will help you retain information in the long term. If you don't think one of the statements will work for you, don't check it. Refer to this list after completing an exam.

☐ Reward yourself. Go for a walk, talk to a friend, get yourself a special treat, or _____ (Fill in something you enjoy doing).

☐ Look up any information that was asked on the test that you couldn't answer.

☐ Once you get the test back, look over your mistakes and make sure you understand what you did wrong.

☐ Ask your instructor any questions that you have about the test to ensure that you fully understand the mistakes you made.

☐ Review any feedback written on the test.

☐ Review your notes periodically.

☐ Review your flashcards periodically, if applicable.

☐ Teach the concept to others who are struggling with the information (this is something that could evolve into tutoring once you've completed the course).

☐ Find ways to integrate the information you learned for the test into information you're learning for the next test.

 Summary

This section has offered suggestions for helping you retain information that you learned for a test. Reviewing your test and reading any feedback given by the instructor are some ways to help you retain the knowledge. The most straightforward way to store this information in your long-term memory, however, is simply to review or use the information on a regular basis.

 Review

Determine whether the following statements are true or false. Select the correct response. Answers are provided at the end of this book.

1. True   False   Reviewing feedback given on a test will help you retain information in your short-term memory, but not your long-term memory.

2. True   False   After completing a test, it is best to spend at least an hour immediately after the test reviewing information that you were unsure about.

3. True   False   Retaking a test is a good way to retain information in your long-term memory.

References

Gettinger, M. & Seibert, J. K. (2002). Contributions of study skills to academic competence. *School Psychology Review, 31*(3), 350-365.

Howe, M. L. & Branierd, C. J. (1989). Development of children's long term retention. *Developmental Review, 9*(4), 301-340.

Jensen, E. & Nickelsen, L. (2008). *Deeper learning: 7 powerful strategies for in-depth and longer-lasting learning.* Thousand Oaks, CA: Corwin Press.

Kang, S. H., McDermott, K. B., & Roediger, H. L. (2007). Test format and corrective feedback modify the effect of testing on long-term retention. *The European Journal of Cognitive Psychology,19*(4-5), 528-558.

Ruhm, C. (1997). Is high school employment consumption or investment? *Journal of Labor Economics, 15*(4) , 735–776.

Stinebrickner, R. & Stinebrickner, T. (2003). Working during school and academic performance. *Journal of Labor Economics, 21*(2), 473-491.

Terry, W. S. (2006). *Learning and memory* (3rd ed.). Boston: Pearson Education, Inc.

Chapter 2: Getting the Most from Lectures

Section 2.1

1. A. Research has shown that most learning comes from preparing for class.

2. False   Most students do not complete assigned readings before lecture.

3. Answers may vary.

Section 2.2

1. True   Research has repeatedly shown that the amount of notes taken during lecture is positively correlated with a student's performance on assessments in that class.

2. False   It is not necessary to write down every detail presented by an instructor in class, especially if the details are directly reproduced in another class resource such as a textbook.

3. False   The majority of university professors use lecture format as their primary instructional method.

4. True   Students should be prepared to take notes before arriving at class.

5. False   Attempts at multitasking in this fashion may result in the note-taker missing key pieces of information. Furthermore, outlining is most effective once all of the lesson material has been acquired.

6. False   It is especially important for students to capture unfamiliar lecture content. This will help them direct their study efforts toward areas of need. Failing to record unfamiliar lecture information because of a lack of initial understanding may result in the student overlooking the content when studying.

Chapter 3: Everyday Learning

Section 3.1

1. False   It is better to study in a cool room.

2. True   Research has shown that it is effective to study under conditions similar to those in which you will be tested.

3. False   The fewer distractions, the better.

4. False   Some people study best in the morning, but others study best at other times of the day.

Section 3.2

1. False   It is a good idea to spend time trying to relate new information to information you already know.

2. True   The more organized you are, the better you will remember information.

3. False   Writing will help your memory.

Section 3.3

1. False   Auditory learners benefit most from hearing information aloud.

2. True   Visual learners like to see the information they are to learn.

3. True   Kolb's model has four categories describing how someone takes in and processes new information.

4. True   Kolb's and Felder's models distinguish learners as either reflective or active learners (and either concrete or abstract.)

5. A. Checking your work is the most appropriate response. This type of learner should make sure time is set aside to review his or her work and not solely trust his or her intuition. Option B refers to a sequential learner, option C refers to an active learner, and option D refers to global learner.

6. C. Taking time to think about your notes is the most appropriate response. This type of learner should make time to think and reflect on new material. Option A refers to a sensory learner, option B refers to an active learner, and option D refers to a sequential learner.

Section 3.4

1. C. Artists are visual learners and tend to picture objects in three-dimensional space.

2. C. Statisticians work with numbers.

3. A. Athletes use their bodies to "solve problems" on a field, such as a basketball court.

Section 3.5

1. True   The purpose of mnemonic devices is to help you memorize information.

2. False   Reviewing facts over a period of time is a much more powerful and productive learning strategy than trying to memorize information in one session.

3. Answers may vary.

Chapter 4: Purpose of Assessments

Section 4.1

1. True   Classroom assessments can be referred to as formative (e.g., quiz) or summative (e.g., final exam).

2. False   Classroom assessments provide information about student performance at the classroom level only, not at the national level.

3. True   Classroom assessments typically include true/false, short answer, performance tasks, and multiple-choice test questions.

4. Answers may vary.

Section 4.2

1. True   The ACT® is an example of a standardized achievement test used to assess how prepared a student is academically to enter college.

2. False   Standardized assessments do not provide information related to a specific course's outcome.

3. True   Standardized assessments provide detailed information about how students are performing nationally, often through the use of percentile ranks.

Section 4.3

1. B. For a standardized assessment, test specifications (such as objectives and content) are typically developed through a formal job analysis procedure. Standardized tests are not usually hand-scored, are not written by the instructor, and are not commonly used to guide instructors' lesson plans.

2. Answers may vary.

Chapter 5: Before the Test

Section 5.1

1. False   True/False questions are examples of recognition questions because you have to recognize whether the statement is true or false.

2. True   Contrary to many people's belief, recognition questions are more difficult than recall questions.

3. True   The question format you expect on a test will affect your test score more than the difficulty you expect of the test. Students study differently, for example, if they know the test is recognition versus a recall test.

4. A. The purpose of the question is to determine if you know how to perform the subtraction.

     B. The question is: what is the solution to 5,432 - 2,345?

     C. The key is A.

Section 5.2

1. True   Your short-term memory stores information that you view for a short period of time and it does not keep the information readily available for the long term.

2. True   It is beneficial to study alone, but it is also useful to share ideas with others who are preparing for the same test.

3. True   Writing study goals is an effective use of planning time because it will help your studying stay focused.

4. False   Creating mock tests is an excellent way to study because it causes you to think critically about the material and is an active study method.

Section 5.3

1. True   Peanut butter is a low-sugar, high-protein snack that is good brain food.

2. False   Reviewing information with peers immediately before a test has the potential to make you unsure of your knowledge; especially if you and your peers disagree on a question. You've come to the test prepared — trust yourself.

Chapter 6: During the Test

Section 6.1

1. False   About 10 million pre-college students struggle with test anxiety.

2. True   Test anxiety can impair a student's ability to solve problems because it limits the brain's capacity to recall learned material.

3. True   Students typically become nervous and worry before an exam, which may affect their ability to concentrate.

4. True   Common test anxiety symptoms were previously identified in this chapter.

Section 6.2

1. Answers may vary.

2. True   With practice, students can learn skills to improve their test-taking knowledge.

3. False   Many students neglect to read the directions before starting a test.

Section 6.3

1. D. Multiple-choice questions are the most frequently used selected-response format in college classroom tests.

2. A. "All" is an absolute word. These types of words tend to make statements incorrect.

3. B. If you eliminate one option, you have 3 to choose from. This gives you a 1 in 3, or 33%, chance of selecting the correct response.

Section 6.4

1. False   Research has shown essay responses containing spelling or grammatical errors are assigned significantly lower grades than are essay responses containing no major composition errors.

2. True   Students should focus more of their time on questions awarded more points because these represent a larger percentage of their overall test grade.

3. Introduction, topic sentences, supporting detail, summary, and conclusion

4. C. If an essay question asks you to outline an issue, you should describe the main ideas, characteristics, or events.

5. B. If an essay question asks you to discuss an issue, you should discuss different points of view.

6. A. If an essay question asks you to analyze an issue, you should break up the issue into individual components and examine each part separately.

7. D. If an essay question asks you to state an issue or fact, you should state it as precisely as possible.

Chapter 7: After the Test

Section 7.1

1. False   Research is mixed in this area. Some research suggests that working does decrease school performance; other research does not find a significant difference in performance between working and non-working students.

2. Answers may vary.

Section 7.2

1. False   Reviewing feedback will help retain information in long-term memory.

2. False   You can write down anything you wish to review, but give your mind a chance to relax.

3. True   It is a good idea to review mistakes, correct responses, and feedback on a test periodically. This will help you retain the information in your long-term memory.